POLYGAMY

THE BASICS

Polygamy: The Basics is an accessible and engaging introduction to the kinship structure known as plural marriage or polygamy. Tailored for general readers and non-specialists, this book distils research findings from evolutionary anthropology, history, economics, political science, and cultural anthropology to survey polygamy's place in human cultural, economic, and demographic developments from prehistory to the present. It addresses questions such as:

- How have perceptions of plural marriage changed over time?
- Where does polygamy fit within human reproduction and family organization?
- What is the pair bond and is it universal or learned?
- Is polygamy a choice and, if so, for whom?
- Is polygamy inherently harmful?

Drawing on global case studies, it endeavors to help readers set aside their own cultural prisms and preconceived notions in order to examine plural marriage in its proper complexity.

Bruce Whitehouse is Professor of Anthropology at Lehigh University, USA. He has conducted anthropological fieldwork in three African countries and is the author of two previous books, including *Enduring Polygamy*. His research also examines social change, politics, statecraft, and transnational migration in sub-Saharan Africa.

William Jankowiak is Professor of Anthropology at the University of Nevada, Las Vegas, USA. He is the author of more than 126 scholarly articles and 12 books, including 7 edited volumes. His research spans a wide range of topics, including urban China, Mormon polygamous families, and the cross-cultural anthropology of drug foods, labor, and romantic love.

The Basics

The Basics is a highly successful series of accessible guidebooks which provide an overview of the fundamental principles of a subject area in a jargon-free and undaunting format.

Intended for students approaching a subject for the first time, the books both introduce the essentials of a subject and provide an ideal springboard for further study. With over 50 titles spanning subjects from artificial intelligence (AI) to women's studies, The Basics are an ideal starting point for students seeking to understand a subject area.

Each text comes with recommendations for further study and gradually introduces the complexities and nuances within a subject.

URBAN ANTHROPOLOGY
Julian Brash

ECONOMIC GEOGRAPHY
Julie MacLeavy, Kean Fan Lim, and Allan Watson

CHINA
Anna Lora-Wainwright

PUBLIC HEALTH
Fiona Sim and Jenny Wright

SENECA
Christopher V. Trinacty

GLOBAL COMICS
Frederick Luis Aldama

CONTEMPORARY INDIA
Rekha Datta

POLYGAMY
Bruce Whitehouse and William Jankowiak

SUICIDE
Matias Gay

ROMANTICISM
Elizabeth A. Fay

LEADERSHIP
Morgen Witzel

HUMAN-COMPUTER INTERACTION
Alan Dix

For more information about this series, please visit: www.routledge.com/The-Basics/book-series/B

POLYGAMY

THE BASICS

Bruce Whitehouse and William Jankowiak

Routledge
Taylor & Francis Group
NEW YORK AND LONDON

Designed cover image: Rokia Whitehouse

First published 2027
by Routledge
605 Third Avenue, New York, NY 10158

and by Routledge
4 Park Square, Milton Park, Abingdon, Oxon OX14 4RN

Routledge is an imprint of the Taylor & Francis Group, an informa business

Library of Congress Cataloging-in-Publication Data
Names: Whitehouse, Bruce, 1971- author | Jankowiak, William R. author
Title: Polygamy : the basics / Bruce Whitehouse and William Jankowiak.
Description: New York, NY : Routledge, 2026. |
Series: The basics | Includes bibliographical references and index.
Identifiers: LCCN 2026018032 | ISBN 9781041045434 hardback |
ISBN 9781041045427 paperback
Subjects: LCSH: Polygamy--Study and teaching | Human behavior |
LCGFT: Case studies
Classification: LCC GN480.33 .W45 2026 | DDC 06.84/23--dc23/eng/20260828
LC record available at https://lccn.loc.gov/2026018032

ISBN: 978-1-041-04543-4 (hbk)
ISBN: 978-1-041-04542-7 (pbk)
ISBN: 978-1-003-62872-9 (ebk)

DOI: 10.4324/9781003628729

Typeset in Bembo
by Taylor & Francis Books

To our wives and families

I watched tears pool over his eyes:

I was that close; he had glimpses

We were that close; we had glimpses.

– Thomas Paladino Presence, 1983

In warm memory and deep appreciation of William Jankowiak (1947–2026)

CONTENTS

FIGURES

INTRODUCTION

WHAT CAN MONOGAMY OR POLYGAMY TELL US ABOUT BEING HUMAN?

DEBATING PLURAL MARRIAGE

Polygamy, also known as plural marriage, has assumed many different forms throughout history. In much of Africa and the Middle East, it has been so commonplace as to be unremarkable. Nineteenth-century Americans, by contrast, viewed the Mormon plural family as barbaric and morally corrosive. This view has softened in recent decades, influenced in part by television series such as *Big Love* and *Sister Wives*, which have become the most public face of American polygamy. These shows depict functional plural families whose challenges and conflicts resemble those found in monogamous households. Their popularity helped temper American hostility toward polygamy and encouraged some viewers to see plural families as less alien and less threatening.

Riding this shift in public sentiment, polygamy's contemporary advocates—as well as some queer theorists—argue that forming a plural family is a matter of personal choice and should be legally permitted. They rightly observe that monogamous families are hardly free of problems, many of them serious. If society tolerates an increasingly wide spectrum of family forms, they contend, then plural families should be extended the same consideration. Their argument resonates with the broader cultural reality that no single "natural" or universally preferred form of marriage has ever existed.

Today, the family in Europe and North America comprises a diverse array of arrangements: single-parent households, blended

DOI: 10.4324/9781003628729-1

families, cohabiting partnerships, unmarried couples, and same-sex unions. As Vice President Kamala Harris declared during the 2024 US presidential campaign, "Families come in many forms." Polygamy's advocates take note of these shifts and ask: if society now embraces so many nontraditional family patterns, why should a thoughtfully chosen plural family still be condemned as unethical or uncivilized? Others argue that plural marriage should be limited to religious traditions with historical precedent, while still others insist that polygamy must remain illegal.

With expanding global migration, these debates are no longer hypothetical. What many Westerners once regarded as an exotic or distant practice now appears with growing frequency in their own societies. As John Witte observes in his book *The Western Case for Monogamy Over Polygamy*, Muslims, Vietnamese Hmong, Native Americans, Mormon fundamentalists, and migrants from Africa, Asia, and the Middle East increasingly arrive in the United States with established plural marriages. Such families present novel legal and administrative challenges involving health care, education, inheritance, and marital recognition. These issues are not unique to the US—Canada and numerous European countries are also grappling with how to regulate and accommodate *de facto* plural families.

The reappearance of plural families in complex modern societies is further shaped by a renewed openness among some educated, affluent individuals who wish to experiment with polyamory and other forms of consensual non-monogamy. Polyamorists (see Chapter 7) argue that monogamy is an artificial constraint that limits personal development. Many, viewing monogamy as dull or restrictive, embrace pansexual or polyamorous identities. This enthusiasm prompts several questions: Do these new relational orientations signal a radical shift in marriage ideals? Or do they represent yet another American-led experiment in alternative family living—one that, like earlier experiments, may eventually retreat to society's margins? If polyamory is simply the latest iteration of plural family life, how widespread is it, and do the challenges polyamorous families face resemble those found in polygamous households worldwide? Our book seeks to address these questions by examining how and why polygamous families have formed, endured, and sometimes dissolved across human history. In the chapters that follow, we explore the emotional, material, and structural dimensions of plural marriage, drawing on historical and ethnographic examples to illuminate the common concerns and recurring dilemmas that shape life in a polygamous family.

PERCEIVING THE POLYGAMOUS FAMILY: HOW HAVE PERCEPTIONS OF THE POLYGAMOUS FAMILY CHANGED OVER TIME AND SPACE?

Interest in plural marriage is currently high in many societies. In countries as different as China and the United States, for example, journalistic accounts and periodic television programs regularly examine women's attitudes toward life in a plural family. Numerous American websites and social media forums similarly debate the merits and shortcomings of polygamous living. Yet despite this steady public fascination, there are remarkably few long-term studies of polygamous communities as integrated social systems that include both men's and women's perspectives. This absence of a gender-balanced, community-based approach to researching this topic has left public discussion of plural marriage dominated by two opposing groups: advocates of the plural family and its most vehement critics. As a result, the images circulating about polygamy are often exaggerated, distorted, or simply incorrect. We still lack rigorous assessments of the emotional benefits and costs that life in a theologically governed small community entails.

Americans' fascination with polygyny is hardly unique. Europeans, too, have long been captivated by the imagined world of the harem. As early as the sixteenth century, travelers to Ottoman Istanbul speculated wildly about life inside a harem filled with beautiful women. The dominant European stereotype—reinforced for centuries—was that the sultan's wives were abject slaves who existed only to serve him in exotic and sexually charged ways. Centuries later, similarly sensationalized—and more frankly moralizing—views have been applied to Mormon fundamentalist communities from the nineteenth century to the present day.

Nineteenth-century anti-Mormon novels often portrayed Joseph Smith as having acquired mystical, hypnotic powers from a wandering German peddler, using mesmerism to entrap women. Tales of cruel "sister wives," despairing suicides, harrowing escapes, and extreme punishments were common themes in anti-polygamous literature. Polygamous wives were described as "slaves to a system worse than death." Such depictions outraged Mormon women, who strongly rejected the idea that they were "pawns of patriarchy." Seeking to counter these accusations and demonstrate women's agency within the plural family, nineteenth-century Utah legislators overwhelmingly supported women's suffrage—believing, quite accurately, that Mormon women would support the polygamous system at the ballot box.

This modern Euro-American anxiety surrounding plural families contrasts sharply with attitudes in Imperial China. Studies of literature from the Qing dynasty (1644–1912 CE) show that elite male authors frequently portrayed polygamous households as utopian ideals, where successful men enjoyed multiple concubines who were beautiful, erotically skilled, and—critically—never jealous. In this literary imagination, polygyny was presented not as perilous or immoral but as a desirable status symbol. (A similar idealization persists today in some Islamic societies, where a man is permitted four wives; see Chapter 1.)

Yet even in China, popular experience revealed the strain such systems placed on family life. Numerous folk expressions implicitly acknowledge the emotional and logistical challenges of plural marriage. One proverb warns: "Best to have three wives: with two they know where you are; with four you are exhausted." Another observes: "Only a saint can balance all his wives; a mere mortal cannot." Despite such warnings, men continued—and continue—to be attracted to polygyny for reasons that include status, economic display, and increased childbearing, though the latter appeals to some men far more than others.

In contemporary China, polygamy has been formally illegal since 1930, criminalized since 1935, and legally abolished since 1950. Nevertheless, many elite men maintain mistresses, a form of *de facto* or "pseudo-polygyny." China's prohibition aligns with legal norms in most East Asian countries. A similar pattern was common throughout much of Latin America, where a comparable institution—often referred to as the *Casa Grande*—prevailed in which a married, typically wealthy, man established and maintained separate households for his mistresses. Regardless of whether a society once condoned or merely tolerated forms of plural marriage, in most modern nation-states such arrangements have become illicit and are now formally proscribed.

HUMAN FAMILIES: WHERE DOES POLYGAMY FIT WITHIN THE FRAMEWORK OF HUMAN REPRODUCTION AND FAMILY ORGANIZATION?

In the animal kingdom, monogamy is rare. Birds cheat, and so do humans, yet many species nonetheless maintain socially monogamous partnerships. Consequently, researchers distinguish between social monogamy—a publicly recognized, cooperative bond often oriented toward child-rearing—and genetic monogamy, which refers to actual reproductive fidelity. In humans, these social and genetic dimensions are typically blended into a pair bond, defined as a strong, selective, and enduring attachment between two individuals that is often, though not necessarily, formalized through marriage. Such bonds involve a psychological and emotional union characterized by trust, mutual appreciation, long-term commitment, and emotional exclusivity, extending well beyond mating or reproduction alone. Importantly, the presence of a pair bond, as a social norm or ideal, does not guarantee sexual faithfulness.

This distinction is important. While social monogamy is found among up to 90 percent of bird species, genetic monogamy has been observed among under a quarter of them. Monogamy of either form is even less common among mammals. Within the mammalian order known as primates, most species reproduce through mating systems involving one male and several female partners (e.g., gorillas) or through a series of brief, opportunistic sexual encounters (e.g., chimpanzees). Only a few primate species, such as the Azara's owl monkey and the fat-tailed dwarf lemur, are monogamous in both senses.

What, then, of humans? Our species stands out in its expressed preference for long-term monogamous relationships. Human marriage occurs in diverse forms shaped by ecological pressures, social norms, and cosmological beliefs. Despite enormous cross-cultural variation, three primary marriage forms recur: polygyny, polyandry, and monogamy. Polygyny entails one man married to several wives; polyandry involves one woman married to several husbands (e.g., the Nyima of Tibet); monogamy historically referred to the union of one man and one woman, as same-sex marriage is a modern practice. The first country to legalize same-sex marriage was the Netherlands in 2001. Since 2001, 22 countries have expanded monogamy to include same-sex couples. Monogamy can also take a serial form when death or divorce leads to remarriage. The medieval Catholic Church, viewing both polygamy and remarriage as immoral, prohibited remarriage on the grounds that it constituted a *de facto* form of polygamy (see Chapter 1).

THE PAIR BOND: UNIVERSAL, OR A LEARNED PREFERENCE?

Some scholars argue that humans are a hybrid species capable of shifting fluidly between pair-bonded and plural-partner arrangements. Although most people live in sexually monogamous unions, such relationships require ethical commitment and ongoing personal discipline. If humans must be vigilant to maintain sexual monogamy, does this vigilance extend to emotional attachment? Might some individuals find greater life-satisfaction in forming simultaneous emotional and sexual relationships with multiple partners? These questions motivate those who contend that humans are not inherently a pair-bonding species.

Evolutionary psychologist David Barash argues that in earlier small-scale societies, polygyny was far more common than monogamy and that sexual monogamy was likely the exception. Over time, demographic pressure from unmarried young men pushed societies toward monogamous marriage norms, even as elite men continued to pursue polygynous mating.

Anthropologist Agustin Fuentes similarly rejects the notion of a fixed "human nature" and views humans not as pair-bonding but as social-bonding animals. Drawing on the work of Barash and Lipton's (2001) book *The Myth of Monogamy*, Fuentes emphasizes that humans, like many mammals, are socially but not necessarily sexually monogamous. Neither Barash nor Fuentes, however, fully consider how romantic/emotional attachment may temper the desire for sexual variety.

Evolutionary theorists also debate why monogamy emerged at all. One influential hypothesis posits that it arose from the need for intensive parental care. Zoologist Eduardo Fernández-Duque and colleagues extend this logic through studies of owl monkeys, concluding that enduring pair bonds arise not primarily from the need for protection but through continuous nurturing, especially paternal caregiving.

Yet anthropologists have found that in small-scale societies—where kin and neighbors routinely engage in allocare—exclusive pair bonding is not essential for offspring survival. As Robin Dunbar notes, this weakens parental-care explanations for the origins of monogamy. Dunbar proposes instead that the pair bond emerged as a defense against persistent male sexual harassment. A woman who aligned with a protective partner reduced her vulnerability, while the man, in turn, gained assurances of paternity. Sarah Blaffer Hrdy concurs that protection mattered, but adds that male investment in offspring—through guarding and caring—was equally crucial. Evolutionary scholars further argue that those who deny the universality of the pair bond overlook cross-cultural patterns of mate guarding, sexual jealousy, and the persistent human difficulty of sustaining passionate romantic love in plural marriages. Even in societies where extended kin are central, individuals frequently experience a strong pull toward forming exclusive emotional and sexual bonds.

Moreover, some assume that because plural families exist, participants must desire them. Yet research consistently shows that many in such families are less than satisfied (see Chapters 2–4), often form illicit pair bonds, or privately identify a "favorite" spouse.

Constructionist scholars—who argue that the pair bond is a strictly social or cultural phenomenon—counter that "favorite" is a relative term and applies only to some plural marriages. Many paired relationships fail to maintain lifelong sexual exclusivity, yet partners manage nevertheless to sustain long-lasting emotional bonds. The constructionists, cautioning against speculative evolutionary narratives, note that the fragility of contemporary marriage—and the growing reluctance to form marriages at all—suggests that humans are not "hard wired" for pair bonding. Humans, they argue, are a socially flexible species capable of thriving in multiple relational arrangements.

They further point to high global rates of sexual betrayal—20 percent of US men and 13 percent of US women, and 57 percent of UK men and 54 percent of women report having conducted extramarital affairs. Extra-pair paternity rates vary widely cross-culturally: from a low of 5 percent among the Aka and 9 percent among the Yanomamo to a high of 48 percent among the Himba. If humans prefer pair bonding, why is sexual monogamy so difficult to sustain?

Constructionists also highlight that anxieties around paternal certainty shift with local sex ratios. When women outnumber men, male commitment weakens; when men outnumber women, males both pursue more sexual opportunities and intensify mate-guarding. This raises another important question: if the pair bond is a biopsychological universal, why are strong cultural norms necessary to enforce it? Essentially, if we humans are fundamentally monogamous, should so many of us devote so much effort to talking monogamy up and ensuring respect for it? Clearly, societies have mythologized and morally justified the pair bond in proportion to the significance they assign it. This cultural elevation may help explain its enduring appeal. Yet the impulse to form an emotionally exclusive attachment with another person appears with striking regularity across time and place.

The apparent paradox—societies simultaneously glorifying the pair bond while also questioning, revising, or even resisting its relevance—poses a challenge that both strict constructionist accounts and some evolutionary formulations struggle fully to resolve.

WHAT SOCIAL DYNAMICS UNDERPIN POLYGAMY?

Besides monogamy, societies may adopt polygyny or polyandry. Polygynous marriage has been widely tolerated but is often constrained in complex hierarchical societies. Among Mormon fundamentalists, for example, demographic realities mean that only a small fraction of elite men can take multiple wives; many young men are left partnerless. This imbalance is less consequential in large, high-polygyny societies where older men marry younger women, birth rates remain high, and a surplus of marriageable women is often maintained (see Chapter 3). Globally, more than 80 percent of people live in monogamous families. Thus, despite its ethnographic frequency and cultural visibility, polygyny is not the most common human marriage form.

Two forms of polygyny exist: sororal (sister) and non-sororal (unrelated) marriage. Non-sororal polygyny is most common. Sororal polygyny, while less frequent, when both are living together as co-wives, is notable for reduced co-wife conflict. Sisters tend to cooperate more, likely due to genetic relatedness, shared offspring interests, and preexisting sibling hierarchies that diminish rivalry.

Polyandry, by contrast, is exceedingly rare, occurring in about 1.1 percent of societies, primarily in the Himalayas and parts of Southeast Asia. It typically involves brothers sharing one wife to prevent the fragmentation of scarce agricultural land. By maintaining a single household, families preserve their estates; dividing land would impoverish all parties. Under these conditions, men restrict their own reproduction for the sake of household survival.

INDIVIDUAL CHOICE AND SOCIAL CONSTRAINT: IS POLYGAMY A CHOICE?

The family is the most adaptable of all human institutions, readily reshaping itself in response to external pressures. Across cultures, there are many ways to form a family, raise children, and transmit cherished values. Shifts in family form are nearly always accompanied by corresponding changes in gender roles—especially restrictions placed on women. Because women are society's reproductive agents, men in many communities are reluctant to grant them what they consider "too much" autonomy. Decisions to enter plural marriages frequently emerge from the tension between personal choice and social constraint, with women disproportionately subject to the latter. Cross-cultural evidence consistently shows that social coercion is a stronger determinant than genuine female free choice in influencing a woman's decision to join a plural family. Even when "choice" appears present, it is usually bounded by material realities and unstated social pressures.

Yet many women do agree to bear the costs associated with polygyny because they and their parents believe the benefits to be greater. Parents may view plural marriage as a means of forging an advantageous economic or political alliance. Women themselves may hope for greater material security for themselves and their children. Contemporary China offers a vivid illustration: a woman on a popular television program ignited national debate when she confessed that she would prefer being a second wife in a Mercedes-Benz to being the sole wife of a poor man. A similar logic can influence women elsewhere to marry into plural unions. In a constrained pool of life-options, polygyny may represent the "best available" strategy—a pragmatic response grounded in self-interest. But agreeing to marry into a plural household does not guarantee long-term marital satisfaction. Women often worry about whether promised resources will materialize, whether co-wives will safeguard or harm their children, whether they will be mistreated by co-wives, or ultimately neglected by their husband.

In arranged-marriage societies, senior generations seek to shape youth through controlling their sexual and marital choices. Here, offspring are reproductive units whose life paths are guided by family interests, not individual preference. In many Aboriginal societies, for example, marriages for young women were arranged through parental negotiation, with girls expected to join a man as his second or third wife. In such contexts, following parental wishes constitutes the normative pattern. Among contemporary Mormon fundamentalists, young women raised in the community are socialized to accept plural marriage. Those with strong emotional ties to their parents typically follow parental recommendations and "freely choose" polygyny. If estranged from their parents, however, these young women often refuse plural marriage—a refusal that usually entails renouncing their religion and leaving the community.

In present-day Israel, polygyny endures in some Palestinian Bedouin communities, though seldom as a preferred option. A major factor underlying the ongoing practice of polygyny in this population is the social marginalization of unmarried middle-aged women. Many such women delayed marriage in pursuit of professional careers and, upon seeking marriage later, found themselves unable to attract a partner because men preferred younger wives. Under these conditions, some women agree to become second wives—not because they desire polygyny, but because remaining single carries an even lower social status. Even women with university degrees and established careers occupy a subordinate position in the household hierarchy when they enter as a second wife.

Overall, women's ability to choose or reject plural marriage is shaped more by economic and social constraints than by a desire for experimental living. Poor, less-educated women are disproportionately represented among those who "agree" to join polygynous households, while women from wealthier families generally avoid such arrangements. This dynamic characterizes both simple and complex agricultural societies practicing arranged marriage.

Does the same logic extend to contemporary intentional communities and individuals who construct plural families within modern urban settings? The short answer is no. Intentional communities and isolated plural families are exceptions driven by religious commitment, ideological vision, or pragmatic interest. Unlike agricultural societies, where polygyny may be an adaptation to ecological and economic conditions (see Chapters 1 and 3), intentional communities are conscious creations organized around specific cosmological or doctrinal principles that justify non-monogamous living. In this sense, Mormon fundamentalist communities are unique: their plural marriage system emerges from the deliberate choices of a population committed to living according to particular values and ideals. By contrast, non-intentional communities reflect adaptive responses to external circumstances that generate normative expectations about how to live.

In intentional communities, from the nineteenth-century Oneida and Shakers to fundamentalist Mormons and polyamorists in the present day, joining a plural marriage has been framed as a matter of personal choice: individuals may enter the community—or leave it—at will. This sharply contrasts with tribal or historical agricultural societies, where polygyny has long been woven into economic survival and kinship continuity.

In sum, material considerations are seldom the primary motivation for joining an intentional plural community. The driving force is more often a quest for meaning—a belief that spiritual fulfillment, moral renewal, or a more satisfying way of life can be achieved within an alternative community. This millenarian impulse lies at the heart of early Mormon identity, and it echoes in contemporary polyamorous groups whose members see themselves as pioneers of new relational forms.

HOW HAVE MODERN STATES RESPONDED TO POLYGAMY?

Polygamy was regulated by some of humanity's earliest known legal codes. In ancient Babylon, the Code of Hammurabi (eighteenth century BCE) explicitly allowed a man to take another wife if his first wife could not bear children. In the modern era, as nation-states developed their own bodies of statutory law, some drew heavily on their dominant religious traditions to determine the permissibility of polygamy, while others relied increasingly on secular reasoning to regulate marriage. Although very few governments have ever legalized polyandry, many have passed detailed laws governing polygyny. Contemporary states can be broadly grouped into three categories according to how they treat polygynous marriage: *permitted, restricted*, or *prohibited*.

Many governments in the first category—those that permit polygyny—rule over majority-Muslim societies. Saudi Arabia, one of the few modern states governed by Shariah law, imposes minimal conditions on a man's ability to take up to four wives. While the Qur'an requires equitable treatment among wives, Saudi law does not obligate a husband to demonstrate his capacity to meet this requirement before marrying again. Other governments have adopted secular legal frameworks that nevertheless remain permissive toward polygyny. This is particularly common in sub-Saharan Africa, where numerous former French colonies adopted elements of the Napoleonic Code after independence while simultaneously maintaining men's customary-law rights to take multiple wives. In some countries that broadly permit the practice—such as Egypt and Mauritania—wives may include a monogamy clause in their marriage contracts, restricting their husbands from taking additional wives.

In the second category, states allow polygyny but only under narrowly defined legal conditions. Several majority-Muslim countries—including Algeria, Iran, Malaysia, Morocco, and Pakistan—formally require a husband to prove in court that he can provide financially for all current and future wives before marrying again. Some require the consent of existing wives as a precondition for court approval. Men sometimes evade these restrictions by traveling abroad to conduct additional marriages. In India, polygyny is permitted only for Muslims, who fall under the jurisdiction of Muslim Personal Law rather than the country's civil marriage statutes.

In the third category, plural marriage is either criminalized or not recognized under the law in many states. These include most Western nations—Australia, Canada, France, the United States—whose legal codes explicitly prohibit multiple simultaneous marriages and occasionally prosecute offenders. It also includes East Asian countries such as China and Thailand, and several majority-Muslim states such as Albania, Tunisia, and Türkiye, where polygyny is legally banned though sometimes informally tolerated. In some countries, such as Côte d'Ivoire, civil law recognizes only monogamy, even though roughly a quarter of all wives in the country continue to share their husbands with other wives. In places with pluralistic legal systems—where civil, customary, and religious legal frameworks coexist—men may circumvent prohibitions by marrying one woman under civil law and another under customary law. If the man does not enter two civil marriages simultaneously, he is unlikely to draw state attention or face prosecution.

Thus, it is inaccurate to claim that polygamy is simply outlawed in "the West" and accepted in "the East," or that it is uniformly embraced in Islamic societies and uniformly rejected elsewhere. Where polygyny is permitted, it is often regulated through diverse and complex legal conditions; where it is prohibited, it may persist covertly in ways that exploit overlapping or inconsistent legal systems.

IS POLYGAMY INHERENTLY HARMFUL?

Perhaps the most debated question concerning polygamy is its capacity to cause harm. Although women in polyandrous marriages may be disadvantaged in multiple ways, discussions of harm overwhelmingly focus on women in polygynous households, and critics routinely cite the vulnerability of these wives as a primary argument against plural marriage. State efforts to regulate or prohibit polygyny are often framed as attempts to protect women and society from its perceived dangers. Critics typically argue that polygyny generates harm at two levels: the household and the societal.

At the household level, they contend, polygyny places women—even those in monogamous marriages—into a structurally unequal position. A husband retains the unilateral ability to take additional wives, while wives have no parallel right. A woman who must share her husband inevitably experiences diminished claims on his time, affection, and resources. She must compete with co-wives for his attention, while her children must compete with half-siblings for paternal investment. These competitive dynamics often produce psychological distress (see Chapter 2) and recurrent interpersonal conflict among co-wives (see Chapter 4).

At the societal level, detractors argue, polygyny distorts the marriage market (see Chapter 3). Each man who takes an additional wife leaves another man without prospects for marriage and, by extension, for achieving socially recognized adulthood. In societies with high rates of polygyny, large numbers of unmarried young men may become socially marginalized. Critics claim that such men are prone to criminality or political extremism and, in Muslim-majority societies, that they may become recruits for jihadi groups (see Chapter 5). According to this line of reasoning, polygyny threatens the foundations of stable social order.

Among Mormon fundamentalists, however, the consequences of skewed marriage markets take a different form. Young men who cannot find a wife typically look outside the community, but "outsider" or gentile spouses often refuse to enter a plural marriage. This refusal produces an acute psychological dilemma for the young man, prompting him to reassess both his faith and upbringing. Many describe a deep sense of personal loss and confusion, ultimately reinterpreting their adolescent years as misguided or even harmful. Yet unlike the political radicalization theorized in some analyses of Muslim societies, the response among fundamentalist Mormon youth is personal: their disillusionment is directed inward or toward their natal community, not outward toward mainstream society.

Defenders of polygyny, when they acknowledge negative consequences, argue that these harms are outweighed by religious, cultural, or demographic imperatives. Many are traditionalists who interpret their sacred texts as sanctioning plural marriage for the moral good of society. African American polygynists, for instance, see plural marriage as essential for group identity and survival in a demographic and political context they view as hostile. In West Africa, polygynists may justify the practice as divinely authorized and socially beneficial. Fundamentalist Mormons view plural marriage as central to salvation and divine command. Across these groups, polygyny is often framed not as an optional arrangement but as an ancestral or sacred practice that must be preserved against perceived cultural erosion.

At the same time, the arguments of critics and defenders alike are often exaggerated and rest on mistaken assumptions about demographic processes and marriage markets (see Chapters 3 and 5). It is certainly true that material and emotional inequality produces significant problems within many polygynous households. It is equally true that wherever polygyny exists, women regularly protest unequal treatment. The wave of memoirs and "escape literature" published by fundamentalist Mormon women in 2008–2009 offers vivid accounts of emotional anguish and repudiation of both their religion and their plural families. Yet we must be careful not to apply double standards when evaluating controversial practices. Much of this literature resembles acrimonious divorce narratives rather than balanced ethnographic testimony and must be interpreted with appropriate caution.

Problems of marital inequity are, of course, by no means unique to polygynous households. Moreover, under certain circumstances, plural marriage may offer women distinct advantages, including economic security, companionship, or relief from the pressures of intensive marital expectations. The chapters that follow offer a nuanced exploration of these complexities and the broader ethical terrain in which plural marriage and polyamory unfold.

HOW SHOULD WE STUDY POLYGAMY?

Scholars have taken many approaches to the study of polygamy, often seeking either to defend the practice or condemn it outright. Our approach differs: we aim to understand polygamy within its various cultural, geographic, and historical contexts, while acknowledging the benefits, challenges, and trade-offs inherent in plural marriage. We encourage you as the reader to approach this topic with an open mind. Doing so requires reserving judgment until you have had the opportunity to learn how people in different times and places have practiced and understood polygamy—and evaluating those practices according to the standards of the cultures in which they occur, rather than your own.

This stance reflects the principle of cultural relativism, foundational to cultural anthropology. Cultural relativism does *not* require abandoning universal rights or moral commitments. Rather, it invites readers to try on perspectives that may initially feel uncomfortable or unfamiliar, with the goal of understanding a system of beliefs and practices through the eyes of its participants. Achieving this perspective is never easy, especially with a topic as emotionally charged as plural marriage.

THE STRUCTURE OF THE BOOK

Chapter 1, "A global history of polygamy," traces the deep evolutionary and historical roots of plural marriage. Beginning with early *Homo sapiens* in prehistoric Africa, we follow polygamy's persistence across ancient civilizations worldwide. The chapter also examines the role of plural marriage in major religious traditions, focusing on Judaism, Christianity, Islam, Hinduism, and Buddhism. From prehistory through the medieval era and into the modern world, we track how polygamy has changed—and how it has been justified, constrained, or transformed across diverse societies.

Chapter 2, "How do emotions affect people in polygamous relationships, households, and communities?," examines the psychological and emotional consequences of plural marriage for wives, husbands, and children. It explores family relationships, mental health, and gendered experiences in polygynous households. Drawing particularly on psychologically informed research among Israeli Arab families practicing both monogamy and polygyny, the chapter analyzes women's emotionally charged reactions to plural marriage across cultures. It evaluates claims about the negative household-level consequences of polygyny and considers the conditions under which emotional distress or conflict is most likely to arise.

Chapter 3, "Who benefits? The material, social, and demographic foundations of polygyny," addresses a fundamental question: How does a society in which plural marriage is common function? The chapter explores how polygyny shapes the distribution of power and resources within households, communities, and societies at large. It examines the demographic factors—population age structure, sex ratios, and marriage markets—that expand or constrain plural marriage. Attention is also given to the relationship between polygyny, divorce, regret, and the material consequences of marital instability.

Chapter 4, "How do they get along? Polygynous household dynamics," focuses on the interpersonal dynamics among co-wives. It considers the balance between hierarchy and equality, cooperation and conflict, affection and rivalry—forces that are elemental to polygynous households. The chapter reviews mechanisms that various cultures have developed to mitigate conflict and promote group harmony. It also analyzes the significance of the "favorite wife" or "favorite concubine" and how favoritism shapes co-wife competition. In many plural families, the struggle for the husband's attention, emotional support, and financial resources acts as a "sleeping virus" capable of disrupting the household unit.

Chapter 5, "Polygyny and inequality," engages with broader societal debates about polygamy's capacity for harm. Is polygyny primarily a response to social inequality—or does it amplify inequality, contributing to discord, criminal behavior, or violence? The chapter examines how polygynous systems intersect with social stratification, male competition, and patterns of conflict. It evaluates popular assumptions, policy arguments, and empirical research addressing polygyny's societal-level consequences.

Chapter 6, "Polyandry," considers the rarest form of polygamy, known as polyandry. This form arises in specific geographic and social settings and responds to specific economic needs. The chapter reviews different varieties of polyandry and how they function. It considers polyandry's origins and its links to the question of shared paternity, as well as the particular challenges posed by living in a polyandrous marriage. It also examines the advantages and disadvantages experienced by women in polyandry.

Chapter 7, "Polyamory," turns to polyamory and contemporary forms of consensual non-monogamy, asking what these arrangements reveal about gender, sexuality, and marriage today. The recent Euro-American embrace of polyamory and "group marriage" represents the latest experimental adaptation of plural living. Notably, these arrangements combine elements of both polygyny and polyandry—multiple male and female partners linked not primarily as reproductive units but as emotional and sexual families. Their successes and failures offer insight into whether humans are, at base, a pair-bonding species. By examining historical poly-families and the contemporary rise of consensual non-monogamy, this chapter situates new research on polyamory within the broader framework of polygamy.

The Conclusion offers reflections on polygamy's evolving role in human societies and considers its possible futures. It synthesizes insights from earlier chapters to address how plural marriage is likely to change—and which dimensions of human sociality it illuminates most clearly.

FURTHER READING

Anthropologist William Jankowiak's *Illicit Monogamy: Inside a Fundamentalist Mormon Community* (2023) draws on six years of immersive residence in a polygynous Mormon community. The study examines the emotional lives of participants as they contend with the demands, expectations, and disappointments inherent in plural family living.

Dorothy Solomon's *Daughter of the Saints: Growing Up in Polygamy* (2004) offers the author's compelling autobiographical account of the polygamous family she was raised in and, later, of the polygamous family she married into.

Irene Spencer's memoir, *Shattered Dreams: My Life as a Polygamist Wife* (2007) provides an unflinching account of the trials and disappointments she faced while living in a polygamous Mormon community in northern Mexico.

Debra Majeed, a scholar of religious studies, interviewed a sample of African American Muslims practicing polygyny and wrote about them in *Polygyny: What It Means When African American Muslim Women Share Their Husbands* (2015). Her account considers plural marriage in a legal and social context where it is highly stigmatized and largely driven underground.

Bruce Whitehouse conducted anthropological fieldwork in the city of Bamako, capital of the West African country of Mali, to examine polygyny in a setting where it was both widely practiced (roughly one in three married women in Bamako was in a polygynous marriage) and culturally legitimized. He documented this research in his ethnographic study, Enduring Polygamy: Plural Marriage and Social Change in an African Metropolis (2023).

The Myth of Monogamy, by David Barash and Judith Lipton (2001), busts the myth that monogamy is "natural" in most animal species, pointing to evidence of widespread sexual infidelity among birds and mammals, including humans. The authors argue, however, that so-called "social monogamy"—that is, durable and reasonably faithful relationships between parents that strengthen childrearing outcomes—has been a hallmark of *Homo sapiens*' evolutionary success.

BIBLIOGRAPHY

Barash, D. and Lipton, J. (2001). *The myth of monogamy: Fidelity and infidelity in animals and people*. Henry Holt & Co.

Jankowiak, W. (2023). *Illicit monogamy: Inside a fundamentalist Mormon community*. Columbia University Press.

Majeed, D. (2015). *Polygyny: What it means when African American Muslim women share their husbands*. University Press of Florida.

Solomon, D. (2004). *Daughter of the Saints: Growing up in polygamy*. W. W. Norton & Company.

Spencer, I. (2007). *Shattered dreams: My life as a polygamist wife*. Center Street Publishing.

Whitehouse, B. (2023). *Enduring polygamy: Plural marriage and social change in an African metropolis*. Rutgers University Press.

Witte, J. (2015). *The Western case for monogamy over polygamy*. Cambridge University Press.

1

A GLOBAL HISTORY OF POLYGAMY

TAKING THE LONG VIEW

The practice of plural marriage is deeply rooted in the human past. This chapter surveys polygamy's role in the evolution and history of *Homo sapiens*, tracing it from the earliest human communities in prehistoric Africa through ancient, medieval, and modern cultures around the world. It also considers the place of plural marriage in Judaism, Christianity, and Islam, as well as other religious traditions. This historical context is essential for understanding the practice of polygamy in the present.

Although many people assume that polygamy has been limited to a small number of cultures or world regions, it could more accurately be described as humanity's default system of marriage. Of the 1257 human societies in a cross-cultural atlas compiled by anthropologists during the late twentieth century, 1052 (about 84 percent) encouraged, practiced, or at least tolerated some form of polygamy. Of these, nearly all practiced polygyny; polyandry was practiced in just four societies. Most of the references to polygamy in this chapter and the following chapters therefore concern polygyny alone; we will examine polyandry separately in Chapter 6.

In the modern era, many European and American thinkers have situated polygamy within an evolutionary process of social and family change leading inexorably toward monogamy. The American anthropologist Lewis Henry Morgan, for example, in his 1877 book *Ancient Society*, wrote that family structure had gone through five developmental stages, with polygyny characterizing the fourth stage (which he labeled "the patriarchal family"). He saw polygamy

DOI: 10.4324/9781003628729-2

as a temporary and unstable form of marriage and lauded monogamy (or "the Monogamian family") as a hallmark of civilized society. Morgan's evolutionary schema had a major influence on the historical materialism of Karl Marx and Friedrich Engels, whose analysis treated all forms of polygamy as outmoded forms of domestic organization. This particularly Eurocentric brand of evolutionist thought, although most historians and anthropologists now reject it, encouraged generations of modern scholars to misrecognize polygamy as a vestigial or exceptional practice rather than as an enduring component of human family systems. This misrecognition lingers to this day.

Many Marxist theories of unilineal social evolution have been disproven or fallen out of fashion, but some elements of the historical materialist approach remain useful. All forms of marriage are indeed rooted in economic forces, most notably the need to organize and reproduce labor power for the household. All forms of marriage likewise entail hierarchical structures—particularly gendered structures—that bolster elite competitions for power and status. By understanding the material foundations of plural marriage (discussed further in Chapter 4), we can better understand why polygamy remains present in human societies all over the world long after many scholars expected it to die out.

This chapter surveys polygamous marriage from prehistoric human communities through ancient, medieval, and modern cultures around the world. It also examines the place of plural marriage within the three Abrahamic religions—Judaism, Christianity, and Islam. In tracing the practice of polygamy through these eras and faith traditions, it refrains both from passing ethnocentric judgment on this practice and from treating it as an evolutionary dead end.

POLYGAMY IN HUMAN PREHISTORY AND ANCIENT HISTORY

It is unclear when marriage emerged as a social institution, but evidence suggests that pair bonds are anchored deep in our evolutionary history. In fact, pair bonding likely predates the advent of early modern humans some 300,000 years ago. Among our hominid ancestors, a progression toward pair bonds may have begun as early as six million years ago, and may have eventually led to the origin of rules of exogamy (seeking mates outside one's kin or cultural network). From these rules, it has been speculated, the first systems of marriage and kinship ultimately developed.

Since the earliest historical records extend only some five thousand years into the past, we know very little about what marriage entailed during the hundreds of thousands of years during which humans roamed Africa in small hunter-gatherer bands. Researchers have inferred from studies of present-day hunter-gatherers that polygamy was practiced by our prehistoric forager ancestors but was most likely rare. Biological evidence supports this inference. Compared to non-human primates, *Homo sapiens* are characterized by less pronounced sexual dimorphism—that is, we exhibit fewer significant physical differences between the sexes than do other species of ape. Because polygynous mating is correlated with sexual dimorphism in non-human primates, it is likely that polygyny was present but not widely practiced over our species' existence as foragers—with the exception of one specific period.

Genetic surveys of African, Asian, and European populations of modern humans offer indirect evidence that polygyny boomed among their ancestors between seven thousand and five thousand years ago. Far fewer males than females were contributing to the gene pool during this period, suggesting that polygyny must have been widespread. During the Neolithic period (10,000 BCE to 2000 BCE), and particularly during the time from 5000 to 3000 BCE, as prehistoric humans undertook a slow shift from nomadic foraging to settled agriculture, many of them organized into patrilineal clans in which descent from shared male ancestors determined communities' kinship structures, marriage and inheritance practices, and political alliances. Some researchers speculate that inter-clan warfare during this two-thousand-year interval must have killed off many males, leading to a population bottleneck that heightened male sexual competition and encouraged the adoption of polygynous marriage. As the bottleneck cleared and sex ratios gradually came back into balance during the late Neolithic period, rates of polygyny most likely declined to their previous low levels. Polyandry was also probably present among foraging populations during this period.

Evidence indicates, moreover, that monogamy had become a widespread pattern in Europe by the Neolithic period. A recent analysis of ancient DNA collected from several Neolithic and Bronze Age burial sites across Europe finds that the percentage of full as opposed to half siblings in the population ranged from as low as 25 percent at one site in early Neolithic Britain to 100 percent at multiple sites in France. Across the sample, 66 percent of sibling relationships were full, a rate quite similar to those of socially monogamous non-human mammal species. Of the half-sibling relationships found in the sample, the majority were paternal half siblings, meaning that polygyny rather than polyandry was the dominant non-monogamous form of mating and marriage.

Even if monogamy was a strong norm by the end of the Neolithic, however, we know that polygyny was common in many of the human civilizations that subsequently arose. Unlike foraging societies, these civilizations were agricultural and sedentary, and their production of surplus grain led to unprecedented levels of economic inequality—a frequent correlate of polygyny (see Chapter 5). Inscriptions show that polygyny was certainly practiced in ancient Sumer at least as long ago as 2400 BCE, and suggest that polyandry may have been practiced as well. In ancient Egypt (roughly 2000–1000 BCE), pharaohs and members of the ruling elite had multiple wives, as did some lower-ranking bureaucrats. Monogamy was the most common form of marriage in these ancient societies, where multiple wives tended to be a privilege of a few high-status men and sometimes served as a man's protection against childlessness if his first wife could not conceive an heir. In Babylonia, the Code of Hammurabi (1750 CE) included an explicit provision for a man to marry a second wife in the event of his first wife being barren. This law also protected first wives against divorce or abandonment due to infertility.

In ancient Greece (750 to 31 BCE) and Rome (750 BCE to 476 CE), it was common for men of diverse social strata to have concubines—women with whom they had sexual relations and who bore them children. Concubines and their children enjoyed lower social standing and fewer rights relative to wives and their children. Slavery was also practiced in Greece and Rome, and female slaves sometimes occupied concubine-like roles. Plural marriage was not allowed, but neither was it criminalized until very late in the Roman Empire, in the third century CE. Monogamy was formally the rule in both societies, meaning that a Greek or Roman man could have only one legal wife at a time, but the option of concubinage meant that both societies practiced *de facto* polygyny.

Similarly, during China's Zhou Dynasty (1046–246 BCE) and Han Dynasty (202 BCE to 220 CE), laws established that while a man could have only one wife, he could have multiple concubines, who were not recognized as wives and had very limited legal rights, making them more akin to the man's property. A man's right to acquire and keep concubines was proportional to his rank in the feudal hierarchy: a lord was entitled to more concubines than a low-ranking officer, for example. Any children born to a concubine were recognized as belonging to the man and his wife, not to the concubine.

Finally, in ancient Mesoamerica, archaeological records show that polygyny was practiced among the Maya during the classic period of their civilization (150–900 CE), albeit strictly as an elite privilege. For Mayan nobles, as with aristocrats and rulers in other civilizations, plural marriage was particularly useful for forging alliances and dynasties.

POLYGYNY IN THE JEWISH AND CHRISTIAN PAST

Some of the earliest prophets and rulers of ancient Israel practiced plural marriage, from Lamech (a descendant of Cain) through Abraham and Moses to the great kings of Israel. A few of the latter had virtually unimaginable numbers of wives: King Solomon, for example, was reported to have had 700 wives and 300 concubines. By contrast, his father King David had only seven wives.

Jewish polygamy was not restricted to the political elite; successful traders often had many wives. Hebrew scripture encouraged the faithful to procreate; polygyny, which kept female marriage rates high, was one means toward that end. Men in Jewish communities were allowed to take multiple wives as long as they could support them all adequately. Levirate marriage, the practice of marrying a widow to one of her late husband's brothers, was another means of boosting rates of marriage and fertility. If the brother had already married, under levirate marriage he became a polygamous husband. A widespread interpretation limited the number of a man's wives to four. Sororal polygyny was expressly forbidden by the Torah, perhaps due to the frictions recounted in the holy book between sister co-wives Leah and Rachel, both of whom were married to Jacob and whose bitter rivalry is a recurring theme in the book of Genesis.

The Jewish practice of polygyny survived the Roman occupation of Judea (63 BCE) and subsequent destruction of the second temple in Jerusalem (70 CE). It continued in the diaspora, but its frequency diminished. Records show that many Jewish women in medieval Cairo drew up marriage contracts expressly forbidding husbands from taking additional wives. Among Jews in Europe, polygyny was eventually banned in a ruling by Ashkenazi rabbi Gershom ben Judah (circa 960–1040 CE). This ruling seems to have been motivated by a desire to safeguard women against marital exploitation and to minimize domestic conflict amid the harsh economic conditions to which Jews were subjected.

Plural marriage existed among early Christians as well, although the practice was seen with increasing disfavor over time. Legal scholar John Witte, in his study, *The Western Case for Monogamy Over Polygamy*, argues that plural marriage's diminishing frequency among Jews and early Christians stemmed from the practice's fundamental incompatibility with Western ideas about family and society. Witte portrays polygyny as highly problematic even among ancient Israelites, for whom it was synonymous with disorder and conflict (Witte noted that "the Hebrew word for a co-wife (*tzarah*) literally means 'trouble'"). The examples of Biblical polygynists such as Jacob, David, and Solomon, he concludes, helped lead Jews and eventually Christians to the belief that their faiths left no room for such a difficult and potentially strife-ridden form of marriage. Many prominent thinkers in the Jewish and Christian traditions, seeing marriage as a sacred union of one husband and one wife "in one flesh," therefore came to suppose a natural law in favor of monogamy. Some Christians believed that Christ had ended—or at least weakened—the Biblical injunction that the faithful should be fruitful and multiply, thereby altering the nature of marriage from a procreative institution to a fundamentally spiritual relationship between two spouses. Saint Augustine (384–430 CE) wrote that polygamy was a natural practice which had been suitable to an earlier age but which ran counter to Christian teachings. By the start of the second millennium of the Common Era, Christians widely believed polygamy as well as concubinage to be incompatible with their faith.

Such beliefs notwithstanding, both the practice of polygyny and robust theoretical defenses of it kept cropping up among prominent Christians almost until the dawn of the modern era. No less a theological authority than Martin Luther (1483–1546 CE), while he generally discouraged polygyny, could not "forbid anyone who wishes to marry several wives, nor is that against Holy Scripture," he wrote in 1524. Luther saw polygyny as at least a preferable alternative to adultery and prostitution. During the same period, John of Leiden, the charismatic leader of an Anabaptist rebellion in the city of Munster from 1534 to 1535 CE, decided to institute polygyny as a spiritual duty among his followers. John, revered by many as a prophet at the time, claimed to have received divine revelation that the Biblical precept to "increase and multiply" was a commandment. He further believed that the plural marriages of Old Testament patriarchs constituted a good example rather than a cautionary tale.

While polygyny was illegal under church and secular law in Europe, its permissibility remained a subject of theological and scholarly debate throughout the Middle Ages and even into the Renaissance. During the penultimate session of the Council of Trent (1545–1563 CE), the Roman Catholic Church felt it necessary—perhaps in response to Martin Luther—to reaffirm monogamy as the only lawful form of Christian marriage. Nearly a century later, the famed English poet and polemicist John Milton (1608–1674 CE) wrote a treatise on Christian doctrine in which he stated that polygyny was not prohibited by divine law and was therefore permissible for Christians. European advocates of polygyny during this period certainly included zealots like John of Leiden, but they were by no means all marginal figures and wild men.

Polygyny had long been a very marginal practice among Europeans by the time Luther, John of Leiden, and Milton lived, and as the modern era began, it became both socially stigmatized and vanishingly rare throughout the continent. Few Christian clerics and thinkers came to its defense, and for most it never even arose as a question. During the sixteenth and seventeenth centuries, as Spaniards colonized the New World, they sought to eradicate the practice of polygyny there. During the eighteenth and nineteenth centuries, as British and French missionaries established a presence in Africa, they sought—with considerably less success—to root out the practice there as well.

Only with the advent of the Mormon faith in the United States during the nineteenth century did the widespread and theologically justified practice of polygyny reappear among Christians of European origin. Joseph Smith's acknowledgment that God wanted the faithful to practice plural family living was not greeted with enthusiasm. Many Mormon officials pleaded that this had to be a mistake and only reluctantly agreed to embrace the newest religious obligation. The mainstream US society's ensuing resentment, moral outrage, and social conflict compelled the Mormons to travel to the western frontier to establish a safe haven. In the process, the idea that the faithful should practice polygamy formed a core component of their social identity. The belief did not result, however, in the majority of nineteenth-century Mormons creating a plural family. It is estimated that less than 20 percent of the Mormon population was able to do so. The Mormon experiment with plural living was undercut by threats from the federal government to use the military to intervene in the Utah territory and forcibly put an end to polygamous marriage there. Today, only a semblance of the nineteenth-century polygamous family exists in scattered small settlements found in the western US, Canada, and northern Mexico.

In the twenty-first century, most Christians around the world see their faith as incompatible with polygamy. As we will see, however, some African independent churches continue to allow (and, in some cases, encourage) polygynous marriage.

POLYGYNY IN THE MIDDLE EAST AND NORTH AFRICA

The Middle East and North Africa constitute the cradle of the Muslim faith, and the practice of polygyny there since the beginning of Islam must be understood with reference to this religion. The relationship between polygamy and Islam, however, is more complex and contested than it is often presented. In the Arabian Peninsula, plural marriage was prevalent and subject to few limitations before the start of the Islamic era in the seventh century CE. Among pre-Islamic Arabs, for whom raiding and warfare kept male mortality rates high, men frequently became the guardians of widows and orphans. Sometimes they incorporated those widows' and orphans' wealth into their own; sometimes they married the widows or orphans as a means of holding onto their assets. When portions of the holy Qur'an were revealed to the Prophet Muhammad following the Battle of Uhud (625 CE), during which Muhammad's followers suffered many casualties, they included this passage (sura four, verse three):

> If ye fear that ye shall not be able to deal justly with the orphans, Marry women of your choice, Two or three or four; but if ye fear that ye shall not be able to deal justly (with them), then only one, or (a captive) that your right hands possess. That will be more suitable, to prevent you from doing injustice.

Muslims have interpreted this verse in various ways over the centuries. Many scholars believe that the verse was intended to protect the rights of war widows and orphans: it permitted a man to marry a girl or woman under his protection, but only as an alternative to exploiting her for her wealth, and it also limited to four the number of wives he could have simultaneously. Despite this verse's historical setting and the issues of unjust treatment that the verse was perhaps meant to rectify, Muslims taking a "textualist" or conservative literal approach to the interpretation of Islamic scripture have used it as a blanket justification for taking multiple wives ever since, whether motivated by their own sexual desire, the pursuit of social status, or other reasons.

Before this verse was revealed to him, the Prophet Muhammad had spent 25 years married to one woman, his first wife Khadijah. In the years following Khadijah's death, however, Muhammad also married ten other wives (most of them widows), often forging new political alliances with the brides' fathers or strengthening existing alliances by doing so. His normative example therefore has encouraged generations of his followers to practice polygyny and has remained a powerful legitimizing factor for polygyny throughout the Islamic world.

While a Muslim basic man's right to marry up to four wives at a time was rarely disputed or even discussed throughout centuries of classical Islamic jurisprudence, Muslim scholars and judges have actively debated how to define the Qur'anic standard equitable treatment of wives within polygynous marriage—more particularly, how a dutiful husband should divide his time, resources, and affections among his wives. Muslim jurists also agreed that wives had a right to marital companionship and sexual fulfillment, though they did not generally specify how husbands should uphold this right, and focused for the most part on how to discourage and punish cases of extreme neglect within marriage.

In the modern era, some Muslim reformists have taken a more critical stance toward polygyny. Muhammad Abduh (1849–1905 CE), a noted Egyptian scholar, notably argued that Muslim societies should abolish plural marriage. Like many early Christian thinkers, Abduh saw polygyny as a practice that had been acceptable in earlier times but that had outlived its usefulness. Some modern Muslims have cited the Prophet's long, contented marriage to his first wife Khadijah, along with his refusal to let his son-in-law Ali take a second wife, as evidence that monogamy constitutes a higher state of marriage to which Muslims should aspire. Such approaches, in opposition to conservative textualist approaches, could be considered "contextualist."

Governments across the Muslim world have taken steps to curb abuses within polygyny, sometimes banning it altogether. Turkiye abolished polygynous marriage in 1926, and Tunisia followed suit in 1956. Many Muslim women's organizations have protested against harms associated with polygyny and demanded the abolition of plural marriage. In most contemporary Muslim-majority countries today, however, polygyny remains legal, though there is considerable variation in how closely governments regulate marriage and how or whether they attempt to ensure that polygynous husbands treat their wives equitably. In countries such as Morocco, Pakistan, and Syria, an already married man seeking to take an additional wife must prove to an Islamic judge or arbitration council that his intended marriage is necessary and that he has the means to maintain multiple wives and their children. Many other countries, however, lack such a legal requirement, and their courts are unlikely to punish or even investigate polygynous husbands for showing favoritism toward one of their wives (see Chapter 4). Rates of polygyny have generally been in decline throughout the contemporary Muslim world, and even as many Muslims see polygyny as a significant part of their religious tradition, many others find it hard to integrate into their modern lives.

POLYGYNY IN SUB-SAHARAN AFRICA

Africa south of the Sahara is the region where polygyny—and, for that matter, humanity—originated, and it remains the region where polygyny is most widely practiced today. Demographic survey data show the highest rates are in West Africa, where it is not uncommon for more than a third of married women in a given country (e. g., 40 percent in Chad, 37 percent in Mali) to be in polygynous marriages. Rates run comparatively lower in Central and Southern Africa (e.g., 19 percent in the Democratic Republic of Congo and Zimbabwe, 20 percent in Mozambique) and lower still in East Africa (e.g., 9 percent in Kenya, 15 percent in Tanzania). It is true that many of the African countries with the highest polygyny rates, such as Mali and Senegal, are also home to majority-Muslim populations. But, with the exception of a few outliers like South Africa (where the polygyny rate is under 2 percent), sub-Saharan African countries have much higher rates of polygynous marriage than do Muslim-majority countries in North Africa, the Middle East, or South and Southeast Asia. For reasons scholars cannot agree upon, polygyny tends to thrive in societies south of the Sahara.

The trans-Atlantic slave trade may have been one factor that shaped this tendency. By comparing present-day demographic data with historical data, economists John T. Dalton and Tin Cheuk Leung found that African communities from which residents were captured and enslaved two or three centuries ago are likely to have a demographic environment conducive to polygyny. Slave raiders working from Africa's Atlantic coast, unlike slave raiders working from the Indian Ocean coast, targeted mainly males. Sex ratios in West Africa, Dalton and Leung hypothesize, remained skewed toward females for generations after slave raids ended, even into the twentieth century. These sex ratios in turn generated a surplus of women in the region's "marriage markets" (the spaces or processes through which men and women were matched as husbands and wives; see Chapter 3), encouraging men to take multiple wives. Dalton and Leung's argument can help explain the enduring strength of polygyny in Africa, as well as why the continent's western region—where most of the victims of the trans-Atlantic trade were captured—remains home to higher polygyny levels than other parts of the continent.

We have seen that polygyny in other parts of the world tends to be an elite practice and/or limited to special cases such as childlessness. In Africa, by contrast, it is far more generalized as a social institution. In the middle decades of the twentieth century, social scientists predicted that polygyny would rapidly fade from African communities as the continent modernized and urbanized. And while polygyny rates have indeed declined in most African countries since that time, the decline has not been nearly as significant as forecast. While polygyny has a stronger economic rationale in rural than in urban communities (see Chapter 4), for many African urbanites it remains a pillar of social and marital life.

Currently home to the fastest rates of urban growth in the world, as well as rapidly growing numbers of educated young people, African societies have undergone significant social transformation in recent years and are poised for much more to come. Amid these changes, polygynous marriage—whether as a practical strategy of domestic organization amid economic precarity, a time-honored custom forged by the ancestors, or a means of pursuing social status—seems to be adapting rather well to Africa's new social and demographic realities. In countries like Mali or Chad, polygyny remains the "normative" type of marriage, and while most married people in these countries are in monogamous marriages at any given time, most of them can also expect to experience polygyny at some point in their lives. Even African Christians are not unlikely to find themselves in polygynous marriages. Mission Christianity's opposition to polygyny proved to be a major obstacle to winning African converts. The rise of African independent churches in recent decades in countries like Nigeria, the Democratic Republic of Congo, and Mozambique has meant a more accommodating stance toward polygyny, which many of these churches' leaders and members interpret as reconcilable with their Christian faith.

Polygyny's place in the social order of African societies has hardly gone uncontested, however. Plural marriage on the continent has in fact faced serious challenges from African women's organizations, socialist states, and most recently, evangelical churches. Many women's groups, particularly during the transition from colonial rule to independence in the 1960s, opposed polygyny less for its inherent injustices and more for the potential for abuse that they believe accompanies it. Socialist states, such as Guinea and Mozambique, once sought to eliminate polygyny in keeping with their egalitarian doctrines and woman-friendly policies; since the 1990s, these countries' post-socialist regimes have largely given up that effort. And evangelical Christians, particularly the fervent Pentecostals whose churches have burgeoned across the Global South, regard polygyny as antithetical to their Christian values and beliefs, a cultural holdover that is essentially pagan, possibly even Satanic. Of the many forces arrayed against African polygynous marriage, evangelical Christianity today is the most powerful, and will surely continue to mount fierce opposition to the practice.

Still, polygyny will most likely continue to thrive in many parts of the continent. It will remain strongest wherever Islam provides it with a legitimizing discourse and protection against Christian evangelization. It will also remain strong in agricultural communities where it provides an efficient system for organizing household labor and production. In cities and towns, particularly where certain churches are seeking to root it out, it is not so much fading away as changing form—becoming more flexible, less formalized, and less rooted in local custom. The structure of polygyny taking the form of separate semi-autonomous households, each of them organized around one woman and all of them united by one man, has been gaining ground in this dynamic environment. The model of polygyny that many African traditionalists have celebrated and advocated, with a man and all his wives and children dwelling together in a single compound, working and socializing as a single unit, has been giving way.

POLYGYNY IN ASIA

Plural marriage in various forms has been rooted in the regions of Central, East, and Southeast Asia for thousands of years. While the Himalayas have been home to the greatest presence of polyandry (see Chapter 6), polygyny remains the most widespread form of plural marriage in all of these regions. It continues among elite Chinese men, for whom it is a means of enhancing their masculinity and signaling their prestige. While the practice of polygynous marriage became more difficult after it was formally outlawed in China in 1929 and in Thailand in 1935, it retains a degree of social legitimacy among diasporic Chinese living in the Pacific Rim.

In her study of polygyny in urban Malaysia, anthropologist Miriam Koktvedgaard Zeitzen described the practice in this setting as "on the fringe of acceptability, a culturally ambiguous domain that is both accepted and rejected, often by the same people, for different reasons." It nonetheless remained somewhat stigmatized, to the point that some Malay men kept their second wives secret from their first wives. In this Muslim-majority society that is also home to a significant ethnic Chinese population, elite women often had to accept the reality of sharing their husbands with other wives, even as they condemned the practice. While the overall rate of polygyny is quite low in Kuala Lumpur, Malaysia's capital, many believe it is gaining prominence there, especially among Muslim men. Koktvedgaard Zeitzen describes the threat of having to share their husbands with other wives as "deeply disempowering" for Malay women, rendering them increasingly anxious about their marriages and households.

POLYGYNY IN THE AMERICAS

In North America, polygynous family life long predates the arrival of Mormon settlers in the Utah Territory. As Pearsall notes, polygyny has deep historical roots across the continent. It ranged from the Apache—small-scale foraging groups of the Southwest—to the pastoral Plains tribes, many of which practiced both monogamous and polygamous marriage. Polygyny was especially prominent in complex chiefdoms and state-level societies.

For example, among the Natchez and Taensa—peoples associated with the Plaquemine and Mississippian cultural traditions, characterized by hereditary elites, mound-building, and intensive agriculture—polygynous marriage played a key integrative role. Elite men often married commoner women, creating alliances that linked social strata and helped bind the society into a coherent whole.

A similar pattern occurred in pre-Columbian Central America. Aztec elites widely practiced polygyny as a form of class exogamy that facilitated upward mobility: commoner women, and by extension their kin, could rise in status by marrying into noble households. This marriage system contributed to a fluid sociopolitical landscape in which rival families could compete for succession and inheritance.

The arrival of the Spanish, who imposed a monogamous marital regime in keeping with their Christian faith, disrupted these dynamics. By limiting marriage to one wife and by privileging the first-born male heir, the imposed monogamous system reduced the number of families eligible to compete for political authority. These changes contributed to the emergence of large, landed estates and effectively reconfigured Aztec society. Within the span of a single generation, this reconfiguration broke the kinship bonds and successional systems that held the empire together, fundamentally destabilizing Aztec political structures.

CONCLUSION

Plural marriage is an integral part of human history. It has been practiced and continues to be practiced in every region of the world. Our survey of its distribution across time and space shows it to be highly variable and adaptive. Polygyny has been by far the dominant form of plural marriage. It has been a privilege of elites in some societies and a more general marital arrangement in others. It has been bolstered by one world religion, Islam, while being largely shunned by two others, Judaism and Christianity. While its frequency has diminished during the modern era, it continues to serve a number of cultural and economic functions. For this reason, this form of marriage is unlikely to disappear, even amid the disruptions caused by globalization and urbanization.

FURTHER READING

Legal historian John Witte's *The Western Case for Monogamy Over Polygamy* (2015) explores the historical and theological shift toward monogamy in Western society. Witte argues that the decline of plural marriage among Jews and early Christians was driven by its fundamental incompatibility with Western ideals of family and social order. Ultimately, he illustrates how these faith traditions came to view polygamy as a source of disorder and conflict, leading to the establishment of monogamy as a central cultural norm in Europe.

Anthropologist Ross Hassig's *Polygamy and the Rise and Demise of the Aztec Empire* (2016) considers elite polygyny a fundamental tool of Aztec political expansion, allowing rulers to forge vital alliances and consolidate imperial power. Hassig argues that the Spanish conquest succeeded not just through military force, but by destabilizing the Aztec social and political order through the forced imposition of monogamy. The book ultimately demonstrates that the shift to monogamy undermined the kinship structures that had sustained the empire's growth and succession.

Historian Sarah Pearsall's *Polygamy: An Early American History* (2019) challenges the notion that plural marriage was a marginal curiosity in pre-Columbian and colonial America, positioning it instead as a central conflict in the development of American social and legal structures. By examining diverse groups—from Native American nations and Catholic missionaries to the early Mormon settlers—she reveals how the debate over "proper" domesticity was used to define the boundaries of citizenship and civilization. Ultimately, the book demonstrates that the sustained campaign by European colonial powers to eradicate polygamy in the New World was less about morality and more about the consolidation of state power and the imposition of a specific racial and religious order.

Women, Islam and Everyday Life: Renegotiating Polygamy in Indonesia (2009) by Nina Nurmila, a scholar of gender and Islamic studies, uses the author's ethnographic fieldwork to examine the lived experiences of Indonesian women in polygamous marriages and the competing religious interpretations that surround the practice. Nurmila critiques "textualist" views that treat polygyny as an absolute male right, arguing instead for a contextual approach that prioritizes the Quran's central ethic of justice for the powerless. Her study concludes that polygamy frequently results in injustice for women and children, suggesting that a truly just Islamic law should favor its abolition.

Legal scholar M.A.Z. Yamani, in *Polygamy and Law in Contemporary Saudi Arabia* (2008), provides an inside look at the resurgence of polygamy in modern Saudi Arabia, exploring how wealth and a return to certain religious values have fueled its popularity among both educated and uneducated classes. Through interviews, she investigates the complex social, economic, and emotional incentives that drive individuals toward plural marriage despite the challenges it often creates for women. Yamani argues that contemporary practice often stems from a misapplication of original Islamic legal principles, influenced by a blend of tribal customs and modern materialistic pressures.

BIBLIOGRAPHY

Hassig, R. (2016). *Polygamy and the rise and demise of the Aztec Empire*. University of New Mexico Press.

Nurmila, N. (2009). *Women, Islam and everyday life: Renegotiating polygamy in Indonesia*. Routledge.

Pearsall, S. (2019). *Polygamy: An early American history*. Yale University Press.
Witte, J. (2015). *The Western case for monogamy over polygamy*. Cambridge University Press.
Yamani, M. A. Z. (2008). *Polygamy and law in contemporary Saudi Arabia*. Ithaca Press.

2

HOW DO EMOTIONS AFFECT PEOPLE IN POLYGAMOUS RELATIONSHIPS, HOUSEHOLDS, AND COMMUNITIES?

COOPERATION, COMPETITION, AND CONFLICT

Polygynous marriage is grounded in intriguing complexities that generate their own kinds of stress, tacit anxieties, and emotional strain. The degree to which any individual is drawn into this complex family system varies with personality as well as the strength of available social and material support.

Researchers have categorized polygynous families into "high-functioning" (cohesive and reasonably harmonious) and "low-functioning" (divided and prone to conflict). In high-functioning polygynous families, there are sufficient financial resources to support all members. Spouses treat one another with mutual respect, co-wives generally cooperate (if sometimes in a more instrumental than affectionate way), and husbands adopt an "enlightened" stance: they are emotionally present, interact regularly with wives and children, and communicate through ongoing dialogue and small, everyday acts of kindness. Among Mormon fundamentalists in particular, a college education for all spouses is a reliable predictor of a more supportive dialogue between co-wives and between fathers and their families, including their wives.

By contrast, in the more common low-functioning families, dissatisfaction typically stems from insufficient economic resources, limited husband involvement, and the presence of co-wives who prioritize their own interests over those of the broader family unit.

DOI: 10.4324/9781003628729-3

Although high-functioning families possess greater material security and demonstrate heightened sensitivity to the complexities of plural household dynamics, this should not be interpreted as evidence that they have resolved the inherent challenges of forming and sustaining a plural marriage. These distinctions—and the dynamics that underlie them—will be examined in greater depth in Chapter 4.

Beyond material and organizational factors, the capacity to sustain a commitment to family harmony depends heavily on how individuals—especially husbands—manage their wives' need for ongoing affection and reassurance. The existential dilemma embedded in the Mormon fundamentalist polygynous lifestyle stems from each wife's yearning to form a more exclusive emotional bond with her husband. These declarations of exclusive love are rarely articulated publicly, but they are visible in daily behavior. The unvoiced desire for greater spousal intimacy is a primary source of co-wife jealousy. The wish for greater exclusivity observed among fundamentalist Mormon women in the United States is not unusual cross-culturally.

As noted earlier, the cross-cultural literature on polygyny is filled with accounts of co-wife jealousy and open hostility. Women tolerate sharing their husbands to varying degrees. Many find some satisfaction in plural marriage when it provides access to a wealthy man's resources or when it offers opportunities to form valued female coalitions. Others frame the arrangement as a test of their personal and spiritual mettle. Christine Brown Woolley, who divorced her husband in 2021 after years being featured among the four wives in his polygamous Mormon family on the television series *Sister Wives* (see Introduction), later wrote that women in her community are "taught to believe that being strong enough to watch your husband marry another woman is why polygamy makes us better people. Anyone who can push down the jealousy that inevitably arises has done some work on herself." This view might be echoed, in regions from the Amazon to West Africa to Southeast Asia, by women who also share their husbands with other wives.

Women's willingness to cooperate with co-wives is significantly shaped by whether there are sufficient resources to provide for themselves and their offspring and by their husband's ability and willingness to treat wives equitably (see Chapter 4). Marital problems and stress intensify when either of these conditions is absent. In those circumstances, family life can fracture into a Hobbesian world of competitive individualism and intense self-serving rivalry.

Researchers working in sub-Saharan Africa, Southeast Asia, and elsewhere report that, although material resources may be distributed relatively equally, a husband's sexual attention (a key source for enhanced fertility) and affection cannot be so easily divided. This unequal distribution often fuels ongoing rivalry among co-wives, many of whom prefer a more exclusive spousal relationship than local norms allow. The struggle to reconcile these twin forces—plural familial love and dyadic, exclusive love—lies at the heart of much of the emotional turmoil experienced by fundamentalist co-wives and their husbands.

The scarcity of time, attention, and resources not only shapes relationships among co-wives but also affects the community's male youth and their sense of security and well-being. Growing up in a fundamentalist Mormon religious community, boys are socialized into a polygamous worldview in which only the worthiest men are deemed fit to marry multiple wives. Yet they also recognize a stark demographic reality: there are simply not enough unmarried women to go around. As a result, young men understand from an early age that their chances of finding a mate are severely constrained. This awareness becomes a persistent, quietly gnawing concern—one that never fully disappears.

FUNDAMENTALIST YOUTH AND THE COST OF PARENTAL REJECTION: A CASE STUDY

Mormon fundamentalist youth readily internalize the community's core values and life orientation. A 22-year-old man summarized his goal as "to live in spiritual peacefulness, marry, have children, have a family, and support that family." This is precisely the ideal that parents in Angel Park, a polygamous community in the southwestern US, seek to instill: raising a "good child" who can fulfill the community's highest objective—creating God's ideal family, the polygynous family. Community members recognize that not everyone has the talent or dedication required, and it is widely understood that many attempts to form plural families will fail.

Youth are acutely aware of community expectations and of the judgment they may face if they cannot achieve this ideal. They take seriously the belief that rejecting community norms means "going to Hell because God has rejected you." When youth gather secretly at night—always away from parental surveillance—the question of whether they want, or feel able, to form a plural family is a recurrent topic of discussion. These clandestine gatherings create an anti-structure or liminal zone, free of formal hierarchy, where drugs and alcohol sometimes mingle with intense conversations about parents' behavior, co-wife relations, the legitimacy of their religion, and the basic question of what makes life worth living.

A middle-aged woman recalls the tension between theological beliefs, parental expectations, and personal desire. She admitted that:

> faithful [sons] were expected to serve their fathers in a humble manner, greeting them by saying things like, "I am here to do your will. What do you want me to do? I want to be a humble servant of the prophet."

Her brother, however, "listened to a deep inner voice that told him that this type of behavior just wasn't right." She notes that however hard their father tried, "through example and scripture, his sons struggled to live the principles of our strict faith."

MORMON FUNDAMENTALIST YOUTH

Community leaders strongly condemn these midnight meetings. In the 1980s, youth developed telephone codes to evade parental monitoring. If a mother answered or listened on an extension, the conversation focused on school clothing; once they were certain that parents were not listening, the youth shifted to planning evening gatherings. In those more conservative decades, the "most grievous sin" for boys was being accused of masturbation or "looking at some girl to lust after her." Some believed that one of the leadership's greatest early mistakes was forbidding dances where youth could socialize. Leaders were so fearful of boys and girls forming romantic attachments that they tried to eliminate opportunities for cross-gender interaction. Weekly sermons were filled with admonitions to avoid social contact. The prophet reminded youth: "You girls and boys know when you do wrong and when you do right. You boys know when you hear the servants of God say to leave the girls alone."

In the 1990s, it was common at church services to hear the leader urge young men to stop trying to date girls and to wait to be assigned a wife. He emphasized that mature men had more resources and more dating experience, so young men should not even attempt to compete for a woman's attention.

Not surprisingly, some youths do become romantically involved with age-mates and want to marry them. When such marriages occur, they remove a woman from the pool of partners available for placement marriage. Angel Park leaders are acutely aware that peer group gatherings threaten the placement system, in which religious elites assign spouses and select a person's "heavenly mate." The community's tacit opposition to male adolescents is closely tied to the chronic shortage of women available to sustain a polygynous system.

This ambience toward unmarried youth is common in polygynous communities worldwide, where "old men often have hostility toward young, unmarried men" and young men are "bursting over with envy and resentment toward the older men in control." A priesthood leader in Angel Park made this tension explicit in a Sunday meeting when he reminded unmarried young men that mature males had more resources and experience and that they should therefore not attempt to compete for women's attention.

Angel Park's tacit intergenerational antagonism over access to females in Angel Park was also common among Plains Indians. Historian Pekka Hämäläinen reports that the more successful some Lakota Sioux men became, the larger the pool of men who struggled to marry at all. "It was a dangerous social pathology that threatened to divide the Lakota men into fully franchised and marginalized individuals." This Lakota pattern continues to be found in most American fundamentalist polygamous communities. It drove the Lakota, and, two hundred years later, Angel Park youth, "to see one another as [more often than not] rivals rather than comrades," in the words of one historian. When the intergenerational competition becomes more explicitly voiced, it signals a disenchantment with the person's belief system, which makes the continued adherence to that system more fragile and suspect.

While the official cosmology demands obedience and respect for authority, many youths openly defy it. A 20-year-old woman in Angel Park, for example, described how she learned to manipulate community expectations. "I learned how to play with my mother," she explained. She and her friends first presented themselves as the ideal daughters their mothers wanted— "nice little girls" who stayed home, had children, and obeyed their parents. Yet, privately, they longed to "go places and do things" and resisted being "fenced in." She admitted that she did not yet know what she wanted but was certain she did not wish to enter a placement marriage. She and her friends secretly drove to nearby towns at night, playing loud music. "We just had fun," she recalled. "Some of the girls would buy beer and cigarettes. We wanted to be bad." Many, though not all, young men engaged in similar acts of defiance.

Philosopher John Saul reminds us that a culture's ideology is, "like theater, dependent on the willing suspension of disbelief. Once the suspension goes, willingness converts into suspicion—the suspicion of betrayal." Although Mormon fundamentalist youth want to retain a strong commitment to their faith, many, especially during the adolescent years, simultaneously harbor a suspicion that the plural family is an institution with serious problems.

The ambience accounts for much of youth's defiance. For others, their defiance is part of the broader adolescent search for identity. One 28-year-old man described his struggle: "The religion did not scare me; in fact, I liked it. For me it was striving to create an identity that was my concern. Where is my place? This question haunts me and my friends." His reflective odyssey is representative and shared amongst community youth.

Unmarried youth often identify with the tortured protagonist in *The Phantom of the Opera*. Like youth in Montana polygynous communities, Angel Park adolescents frequently turn to alcohol and illegal drugs to cope with anxiety.

MORMON FUNDAMENTALIST SOCIAL HIERARCHY

Fundamentalist youth who are from a low-ranking family are seldom given a wife; thus, most leave the community to find a mate, who inevitably refuses to join which inevitably results in her refusal to move to the polygamous community. Once a youth has left the community, there is a revision in how they conceptualize their childhood. Having an intimate understanding of the plural family's difficulties, they come to define themselves in opposition to the community's faith-based norms. However, when a youth comes from an elite family, or part of an elite family, he recognizes that he will indeed be assigned a mate and tends to be less drawn to leaving the community.

The ability of elite families to hold on to their sons results in "clan cannibalism," whereby elite males attract daughters from non-elite families who prefer to marry into the more elite families. This pattern of incorporating low-ranking females into higher-ranked families over time results in the high-ranking families becoming, in the words of two anthropologists, "larger, more powerful, and to reproduce more successfully overtime, while low-ranking families ... become smaller, less powerful, and reproduce less successfully."

Whatever the quality of a youth's home life or his father's social rank, there are other social structural factors that contribute to a limited marriage market. It is telling that the community adopts a blind eye to this reality: the shortage of females. In avoiding the structural deficiency inherent in a plural family system, the community finds solace in its nineteenth-century metaphysical perspective, which ascribes a young man's inability to find a mate to his lack of character or weak moral fiber. It is this idea that youth have internalized that contributes to their feeling of acute personal inadequacy.

For the community, the youth who leave represent God's rejection of them as suitable candidates for living in "God's chosen community." In the common parlance of the community, a youth is either a "good" person or a "Devil" person. The distinction is common in many fundamentalist communities, which habitually, constantly, draw lines between the "elect" and the "damned" or unsaved. A youth's departure is regarded as a simple example of one "losing the spirit of the Lord" and therefore "losing the spirit of the Work."

Females, in contrast, have no worries about finding a spouse. They are concerned about the quality of their future husband—whether he is a decent man and not too old. Certainly, this does not mean that some females do not have occasional existential doubts about the viability and suitability of forming a plural family. Unlike males, however, they have a certain safety: if they ever leave the community, they can always return and be immediately honored for doing so. Nonetheless, many females struggle with the existential decision to stay or leave. A few of them admit having been "wild" as teenagers and, in their words, "sinned often."

Some girls will leave the community and take up with a boyfriend, drink in excess, and, surprisingly, join in sex parties, only to discover in their early twenties that they truly belong in the community and that leaving was a mistake. For example, one young woman wrote a letter to her mother praising the polygamous family, admitting she came close to being damned but now wishes to return to become a plural wife, stating that she feels refreshed and fulfilled in the prospect of doing so. She thanked her mother for her love and for never abandoning the hope that she would return. In Angel Park, prodigal daughters are warmly invited back and immediately placed in another family. There is less desire, less willingness, to accept youthful prodigal sons, who, unable to find a wife from the community, must thus go outside it, seldom returning.

INTERGENERATIONAL TENSION

The demographic realities in this community ensure there will always be a skewed ratio of more males wanting a wife than there are potential wives available (although the problem is different in other social settings, as we will see in Chapter 3). This skewing further accounts for young males' acute anxiety over whether they can marry and thus remain in the community. It is this sociological factor that leads youth to engage in serious, often internal reflection on the viability of their religion. As a result, successful adolescence socialization depends upon more than effective parent-child interaction, a necessary but insufficient condition for producing what the community deems its major spiritual and cultural ideal: the production of men and women capable of forming— not only capable of but in fact forming—a plural family.

Young women face no shortage of suitors; their concern centers on the *quality* of a future husband—whether he is decent and not too old. Some do experience existential uncertainty about plural marriage, but unlike young men, they have a built-in safety net: a woman can always return to the community and be immediately honored for doing so. Still, many female adolescents struggle with whether to stay or leave. Prodigal sons who leave face a different fate. Having left because they could not obtain a wife inside the community, they seldom return. When they do, it is typically in middle age or later, and any marriage they obtain is usually with a postmenopausal widow who seeks a protector and benefactor. Their reintegration lacks the celebratory quality extended to returning daughters.

Every family, in its own way, strives to raise children as "good" persons and must navigate more than simple adherence to doctrine. The demographic realities of the plural family system ensure a permanently skewed ratio: more males seeking wives than there are potential wives available. This imbalance produces deep anxiety among young men over whether they will ever marry and thus remain in the community. It is this sociological feature—rather than individual failings—that often leads youth to question the long-term viability of their religion. Ultimately, successful adolescent socialization requires more than effective parent–child relations. While necessary, that relationship is insufficient to guarantee the community's central spiritual and cultural ideal: producing men and women who not only accept but form a plural family.

Regardless of outlook, the central issue facing adolescent males is whether there will be an eligible woman available for marriage. In contrast to Mali and other African societies that practice polygyny and benefit from demographic conditions that produce a surplus of women in the marriage market, fundamentalist Mormons live in small, often insular communities that intermarry among themselves. Some communities have practiced first cousin marriage, which others consider incestuous and taboo. A recurrent concern in these communities is whether there are enough marital appropriate women to sustain plural marriage. The sex ratio distortion provokes amongst fundamentalist youth an acute anxiety over their "righteousness" and "worthiness." It is a never-ending anxiety that promotes emotional distraught and, for some, acute depression that seems to never go away.

THE ISSUE OF EMOTIONAL HEALTH

It has frequently been argued that polygyny can be psychologically harmful. A study of Palestinian women, for example, found that those in polygynous marriages reported more mental health problems than Palestinian women in monogamous marriages. Across multiple settings, wives in polygynous households face an elevated risk of depression and other mental health challenges.

Arab and fundamentalist Mormon co-wives often struggle with a combination of psychological, physical, and social difficulties as they adjust to their husbands' remarriage. This cluster of symptoms has been described as the "first wife syndrome." As one Mormon fundamentalist mother warned her daughter on the eve of the daughter's marriage as a second wife, "You will be better off as a second wife—you will never have to experience the pain of learning to share your husband."

A deep-seated sense of anxiety often emerges among co-wives as they compete for access to their shared husband. During the early years of marriage, co-wife conflict is pervasive and can be marked by episodes of verbal and even physical violence. Cross-cultural research shows that most women react to the arrival of a new co-wife with fear, anger, sadness, and a sense of loss. These sentiments are expressed through a range of culturally recognized behaviors: witchcraft accusations; concern for the welfare of one's children; accusations of favoritism; demands for increased access to the husband; complaints about being sexually ignored; physical or verbal assaults; and threats of, or actual, divorce.

DO CO-WIVES FORM EMOTIONALLY SUPPORTIVE FRIENDSHIPS?

An issue that also arises in plural unions—particularly among contemporary polyamory practitioners—is liminality: the experience of living in a social "borderland" of respectability. This liminal status can take a personal toll on well-being. Families with children worry about stigma and possible ostracism for pursuing a lifestyle that mainstream culture does not support.

Those who seek counseling often find that therapists are unprepared to respond effectively to the unique challenges of complex non-monogamous families. Others, however, report that counseling has been helpful and has improved the emotional quality of their relationships. For them, the plural love bond is not simply a source of strain but can make life feel deeply meaningful.

In non-Western settings, there are also examples of co-wife relationships that become genuinely supportive. In some societies, a middle-aged woman without children may negotiate with a younger woman who agrees to care for her in old age in exchange for the older wife's support and non-interference in the marriage. Such arranged co-wife relationships can be relatively cooperative, less stressful, and mutually beneficial. Elsewhere, subsistence demands require co-wives to work closely together. These shared tasks sometimes foster deep friendships that endure into old age. In such cases, women's special bonds can significantly enhance their psychological well-being. Yet such supportive relationships among co-wives are generally the exception to the rule (see Chapter 4).

STRESSFUL LIVES AND MEN'S HEALTH

Even in settings where consensual non-monogamy is broadly accepted, the pressures created by complex family living affect mental and physical health. The creation of a plural family does not guarantee life satisfaction for either men or women.

Nevo, Al-Krenawi, and Yuval-Shani's studies of Palestinian families found that polygynous women experienced more mental health problems than their monogamous counterparts. A cross-cultural literature review finds that wives in polygynous households face higher rates of depression and other mental health difficulties; the cluster of psychological, physical, and social problems that Arab women experience when their husbands remarry is again described as "first wife syndrome." Across societies, polygynous husbands frequently report feeling "stressed out" by the need to meet their family obligations. Some Senegalese husbands, for example, worry that they are losing years off their lives from the strain produced by wives' physical and spiritual battles with one another. Other research from Saudi Arabia and the United Arab Emirates, where polygyny is legal, indicates that polygynous men have higher blood pressure, higher rates of diabetes, and a greater incidence of coronary artery disease than monogamous men. These men shoulder persistent financial burdens and an ongoing emotional toll as they attempt to care for large and growing households. The cumulative effect of daily pressures on men's health is rarely discussed, yet wives are keenly aware of the strain their husbands endure and often acknowledge the "unbearable" pressure men feel while trying to support their families both materially and emotionally.

Studies also show that Arab children from polygynous families are more likely to suffer from psychological problems and poor school performance than children from monogamous families.

Western-based psychological research has demonstrated that emotional intimacy is a strong predictor of health and happiness. Individuals who are uncomfortable with intimacy or commitment are prone to discontent and dissatisfaction with life. This pattern also holds among fundamentalist Mormons. One common response to the daily anxieties embedded in plural living is excessive drinking. In some fundamentalist communities, alcohol consumption—which is prohibited by the Church of Jesus Christ of Latter-Day Saints—is widespread. Some men drink in their workshops; others over-consume when they come home. Irene Spencer, from the LeBaron community in Mexico, recounts how her husband tried to manage his emotions through heavy drinking, noting that he often drank "before he came to see any of us." Another common response is withdrawal into solitude, as men avoid day-to-day family issues, requests, disappointments, and long-standing problems. Overwhelmed husbands may tell their wives to "work it out among yourselves" and to "leave me alone."

Many men experience an acute existential struggle as they strive to achieve their exalted goal: creating a harmonious, highly functional plural family. Husbands, more often than wives, experience intense guilt or shame when they cannot uphold the community ideal of equal treatment for all wives. Feelings of shame increase among men who take their ethical responsibilities seriously but still fail to provide adequate financial and emotional support to their families. Given these constraints, it is reasonable to assume that accumulated stress profoundly affects men's health and well-being.

WHAT ABOUT POLYAMORY RELATIONSHIPS?

The fundamentalist Mormon ideal of "plural" or multiple love bonds bears a family resemblance to the contemporary cultural phenomenon of polyamour (polyamory)—the desire and capacity to love more than one person—now found across the globe (see Chapter 7). In both systems, participants strive to avoid forming emotionally exclusive dyads. Ideally, everyone in the family takes pleasure in one another's well-being and finds joy in witnessing others' love. For fundamentalist Mormons, however, this is an ideal seldom realized in everyday life.

Successful polyamorous unions tend to be grounded in material affluence and a shared commitment to ongoing, informal conversations. In practice, many polyamorous households function like ad-hoc therapeutic groups. When three or more partners gather to talk about their relationships and the benefits of their mutual love, they engage in a kind of group reflection that can sustain the union. This union appears to not be representative, but more of an aspirational ideal. The typical formation, although not necessarily the preferred union, is to form an emotional hierarchy where one partner is deemed primary.

Unlike monogamous couples, polyamorists report a distinct set of challenges associated with sustaining plural relationships. One of the most significant is the psychological burden created by public disapproval and stigmatization. Additional interpersonal difficulties include managing the jealousy that may emerge within plural arrangements, as well as the anxiety and stress involved in coordinating partners who may live in different geographical locations—making it difficult to ensure that each relationship receives adequate time and attention. When childcare responsibilities are added to this already complex relational landscape, the stressors can multiply further.

By contrast, the question of reproduction and childcare poses few structural problems for most polygynous families. Each wife focuses primarily on her own children, and co-wives seldom have the time or opportunity to engage in regular, in-depth conversations with one another or with the husband. In these settings, attention tends to center on one's natal family.

Polyamorous relationships demand something different: a strong dedication—or even conscious determination—to maintain simultaneous, but separate, life histories or narratives. For some, this is too difficult to sustain. The deliberate construction of distinct personae for different partners can lead to behaviors and feelings associated with a "dual personality," which can, over time, produce inner turmoil. Maintaining several emotionally significant relationships may initially satisfy needs for passion and companionship, but this configuration can evolve into an acute psychological dilemma that some find profoundly dissatisfying and even destructive.

The core difficulty lies in reconciling two types of love: one grounded in intense passion and another based in deep companionship. Elevating one partner as the "primary" or more emotionally exclusive lover while designating others as "secondary" can create chronic tension. Love's pull toward dyadic exclusivity ultimately transforms many, though not all, plural arrangements into enduring friendships rather than truly bonded dyadic units.

POLYAMORY FAMILIES AND PERCEIVED THREATS TO CHILDREN

As noted above, studies of Arab children from polygynous families suggest that they are more likely than children from monogamous families to experience psychological problems and poor academic performance than children from monogamous families. Among fundamentalist Mormons, attitudes toward education vary considerably. More orthodox families often avoid public education, while more liberal or "open to the world" families encourage their children to excel in school. The preferred parenting style is strict and authoritarian, with a ready use of corporal punishment.

In contrast, polyamorist parents who are mostly college-educated professionals prefer discussion and the use of "time outs" over corporal punishment. Sociologist Elizabeth Sheff, whose research focused primarily on how children respond to polyamour parents, found there were few psychological issues (see Chapter 7). As adults, most children recalled with fondness their involvement with multiple adult caretakers. Some reported it contributed to an expansion of life possibilities which further enriched their lives.

Sheff's findings are further supported by anthropologists working in small-scale societies where numerous caretakers are involved in caring for local children. In these societies the children feel emotionally grounded and secure, which contributes to their overall well-being. It is reasonable to assume that multiple polyamorist caretakers would have a similar outcome.

CONCLUSION

The psychological impact of living in a plural family varies by gender, age, and relative material wealth. As we have seen, complex families—whether polyamorous, polyandrous, or polygynous—are not free of structural tensions, psychological conflicts, and challenges to personal fulfillment. The emotional costs common to plural families tend to affect women and men differently. Men's anxiety typically stems from their inability to be adequate providers. The capacity to financially support one's family is a defining attribute of masculinity; when men fall short, feelings of inadequacy, guilt, and shame often follow. In contrast, women's emotional distress arises primarily from insufficient attention from their husbands and the inability to secure adequate material resources for their children. Some women build cooperative, mutually supportive relationships with co-wives, which can enhance their well-being; others struggle to do so and instead rely more heavily on their children and natal kin as the main source of emotional support. Children in plural families, however, often benefit from having multiple caregivers who can provide emotional attention and serve as alternative role models. Exposure to a wider range of behavioral styles can offer a richer nurturing environment in which to grow and develop.

FURTHER READING

Christine Brown Woolley's *Sister Wife: A Memoir of Faith, Family, and Finding Freedom* (2025) is typical in some ways of a sizable "escape literature" written by Mormon wives who have left polygynous marriages and chosen to share their critical insider perspectives on plural marriage with a wider public. Perhaps unique in Woolley's case, however, is the fact that her then-husband Kody Brown's polygynous household was the subject of the long-running reality TV series *Sister Wives*, which first aired on the TLC network in 2010 and was still in production 15 years later. Woolley's memoir is especially memorable for its examination of the intersection between polygyny, celebrity, and media in American culture.

Janet Bennion's anthropological study *Women of Principle: Female Networking in Contemporary Mormon Polygyny* (1998) focuses on how women experience life in a Montana Mormon fundamentalist polygynous community. Rather than passive subjects, women emerge as active agents who define, soften, and reshape what it means to live within a patriarchal social order.

BIBLIOGRAPHY

Bennion, J. (1998). *Women of principle: Female networking in contemporary Mormon polygyny*. Oxford University Press.

Woolley, C. B. (2025). *Sister wife: A memoir of faith, family, and finding freedom*. Gallery Books.

3

WHO BENEFITS?

THE MATERIAL, SOCIAL, AND DEMOGRAPHIC FOUNDATIONS OF POLYGYNY

CHOICE VERSUS COERCION

Over the years, scholars—including many evolutionary biologists and economists—have argued that polygynous marriage serves women's interests by enabling unmarried women to select wealthier husbands who happen to be already married. The most successful males, by this argument, make the best (or, in evolutionary terms, "fittest") potential husbands and therefore attract multiple wives. This argument assumes, as psychologist David Barash has put it, that "sex is something that men purchase and women sell (or are coerced into providing)," and that "the higher a man's status and the greater his wealth, the more likely he is to have obtained more than one wife." This is the same logic expressed by playwright George Bernard Shaw, who in 1903 wrote that "the maternal instinct leads a woman to prefer a tenth share in a first-rate man to the exclusive possession of a third rate one."

In the twenty-first century, similar notions continue to circulate inside the so-called "manosphere," the online environment shaping the gender ideologies of mostly younger men in mostly wealthy, English-speaking countries. Within this space, men talk about being "red-pilled" (i.e., awakened to the many supposed ways that males are disadvantaged in modern society) and categorize all males as either "alpha" (fit, attractive, economically and evolutionarily successful; destined to dominate women and other men) or "beta" (unattractive, unsuccessful; destined to be dominated). "Polygyny is

DOI: 10.4324/9781003628729-4

nature's equilibrium, and we're going back there because it's a better proposition for women than being with a beta," one such "red-pilled" individual in Britain told a journalist. The argument that polygyny enables women to opt for a lesser share of the most successful male mates is sometimes called the "female choice model" (a subject to which we will return in Chapter 5).

Skeptics, including many anthropologists, have pointed out that the female choice model rests on the expectation that women can freely choose their husbands within an efficient marriage market (the spaces or processes through which men and women are matched to one another through marriage). This expectation is hard to justify across times and places. Until the twentieth century, marriage formation in most societies was the prerogative of kin groups rather than individuals. Elders in many cultures today continue to arrange marriages for their children or dependents to form a union advantageous to the group—and particularly advantageous to the male elders who exercise authority over the group and who do not necessarily take the preferences of prospective brides or grooms into account. In short, even in the twenty-first century, the people doing the "shopping" in a marriage market and making the decisions are frequently not the prospective brides and grooms at all, though they claim to be acting in the best interests of the brides and grooms.

Nor, as we shall see, are polygynous husbands unfailingly or even predominantly high-status, wealthy men. Senior men in various societies arrange marriages for their dependents by acting in their own interest, selecting spouses according to criteria that may have little or nothing to do with their social standing or purported "fitness," and preventing junior women (and sometimes junior men) from making any choices at all. Moreover, women often express reluctance to share their husbands with other wives, and many only do so as a last resort. Accordingly, some scholars have proposed a "male coercion model" to better explain polygyny's advantages and identify who collects them. By rejecting the assumption that marriage decisions are made by individual participants pursuing their own individual desires in efficient markets, the male coercion model departs from the female choice model's perspective on polygyny as a natural consequence of inequality among males.

Still, the question of who benefits from polygyny remains unsettled, as the male coercion and female choice models by no means exhaust the possibilities. In the sections to follow, we review various explanations of polygyny's differential advantages. How one thinks about the gains from polygyny stems in part from one's unit of analysis. Polygyny might be seen to work in favor of individual men or individual women; it might also be seen to benefit a household, a community, even an entire population. But none of these units is "objective," and an analysis based upon any of them entails assumptions of its own. For these reasons, questions about polygyny's supposed advantages are best accompanied by the question, "who benefits, and at whose expense?"

REPRODUCTION AND PRODUCTION

Polygyny's unequal advantages become clear when we consider reproduction. One might presume that polygyny leads to more children being born, and indeed, birth rates tend to be higher in polygynous societies than in non-polygynous ones. When we differentiate by sex, however, we find that polygyny only advantages men in this respect, and that women in polygynous marriages have *fewer* children on average than their monogamous peers. Polygyny's effects on population-level birth rates, demographers have discovered, are indirect: since high levels of polygyny are also associated with women's and girls' early marriage, polygyny boosts a population's fertility rate by helping to maximize the married portion of the female population. If having a large progeny is an advantage, as evolutionary theory dictates, then polygyny certainly benefits husbands—at their wives' expense. As Barash has put it, "when a man decides to take a second wife, this is nearly always bad news for the first one." We saw in Chapter 2 that this is true in a personal sense with respect to the first wife's mental health, but it is equally true in an evolutionary sense with respect to her diminished prospects for reproductive success. Polygyny's sharply divergent outcomes by gender lead some scholars to see it more as a function of male coercion than female choice.

Even if we recognize high aggregate birth rates as an advantage of polygyny, moreover, they do not always translate into larger progenies. Several studies found that infants in high-polygyny communities in present-day Africa face a survival disadvantage, even if their mothers are monogamous. For example, one longitudinal survey of child mortality in Mali, West Africa, found that children living in extended family households characterized by frequent polygyny were more likely to die than children in households with less frequent polygyny, irrespective of whether these children's mothers were in polygynous unions. This suggests that in settings characterized by scarce resources, polygyny may heighten intra-household competition, leading to "resource dilution" that stunts children's growth and imperils their survival. Such evidence has been used to support calls for restricting or even abolishing polygyny in countries where it is practiced (see Chapter 5).

Other scholars, however, have questioned whether a clear causal mechanism links child survival to polygyny. They point out that selection into polygynous marriages in the modern African societies under study is not random, since women who enter polygynous marriages tend to be of lower status to begin with, compared to women who enter monogamous marriages. If polygyny disproportionately attracts poor and marginalized women, then poorer child survival outcomes in high-polygyny households may have little to do with polygyny itself, and polygyny may entail no intrinsic disadvantages to children.

Leaving human reproduction aside, for now, we must also consider how polygyny might benefit *economic* production. In 1970, economist Esther Boserup proposed that high rates of polygyny in sub-Saharan Africa were a function of the sexual division of labor necessitated by labor-intensive agriculture. Where farming systems relied on hand tools instead of plows, women often provided the bulk of agricultural labor. A polygynous farmer could therefore profit from his wives' work in the fields; his household could farm more land and reap more harvests. Boserup hypothesized that polygyny is highest in societies where women contribute significantly to agricultural production, and lowest in societies in which women do less agricultural labor. Under this scenario, polygyny's benefits once again go largely to the husband who enjoys the fruits of his multiple wives' toils.

Using surveys from a variety of cultures to show that no strong correlation existed between polygyny and women's role in farming, anthropologist Jack Goody challenged Boserup's hypothesis.

He argued that polygyny stems more from men's pursuit of status, sexual variety, and progeny than from the need for agricultural labor. In short, he concluded, polygyny confers no necessary advantages to production, and therefore the "reasons behind polygyny are sexual and reproductive rather than economic and productive."

It is possible, however, that polygyny offers economic benefits outside the realm of farm labor. Research has posited that polygynous households could be better than monogamous ones at obtaining vital resources such as food or money. A polygynous family in a drought-prone region, for example, might command more potential sources of extra-household support and "risk insurance" via the kin networks of its multiple wives than a monogamous family does. This would make the polygynous family more resilient to the shocks generated by its uncertain environment—an advantage that might help explain polygyny's durably high prevalence in Africa's arid Sahel region. Economists have also hypothesized that polygyny helps households allocate resources among their members more efficiently, but evidence from game experiments conducted in various African communities has thus far offered little confirmation of this. Polygyny is by no means a reliable asset to intra-household cooperation, however: one study of women experiencing health crises in urban Mali found that while they could usually count on support from their daughters and other female kin, they received little help from co-wives.

Another possible advantage is that polygyny enables households to allocate domestic labor more efficiently. Several studies have indeed found widespread labor sharing among co-wives. In Senegal, for example, wives in monogamous households spent eight more hours per week than their counterparts in polygynous households on domestic chores, after controlling for other factors such as age, education, and rural or urban residence; in nearby Mali, urban co-wives relied less on hired or child labor than their peers in monogamous marriages. Kipsigi women in Kenya expressed favorable views of polygyny due to its capacity to supply cooperative labor. In apartheid-era South African cities, Black women described labor sharing with their co-wives, particularly for childcare, as polygyny's greatest advantage; this advantage was especially strong in cases of sororal polygyny (in which sisters share a husband), which historically has been common among the Zulu.

Similarly, in an Aboriginal Australian community where nearly half of polygynous marriages were sororal, co-wife cooperation was found to be strong.

But if labor sharing constitutes a clear *potential* benefit of polygyny, it is by no means always present in polygynous households. Labor sharing is harder to find, for instance, in many urban settings from Africa to Southeast Asia where co-wives express a strong and growing preference to live separately from one another, sometimes even in different neighborhoods. Likewise in rural African communities, as many as 90 percent of polygynous unions can be noncoresidential, meaning that co-wives do not live together and cannot easily help one another with domestic tasks. Some communities, such as the Ga people of Ghana, have a longstanding cultural preference that a polygynous husband house his wives in separate locations. And even in cases of coresidential polygyny, some research has found no significant labor savings for co-wives.

By now it should be apparent that polygyny confers no general, consistent advantages with respect to human reproduction or economic production. The broadest advantage seems to be that polygynous husbands have more descendants on average than monogamous husbands. Even this outcome, however, can be undercut when conditions of poverty lead to higher rates of child mortality in polygynous households.

POWER, STATUS, AND GENDER

At least for men, polygyny is widely understood to be linked to social status, and scholars often frame polygynous marriage as a privilege of wealthy males. Yet the relationship between polygyny and wealth is ambivalent. In African societies, for instance, there is no clear link between men's socioeconomic status or education and their participation in plural marriage. Having multiple wives remains a goal to which African men of diverse social categories—rural and urban, educated and uneducated, high and low status, Muslim and Christian—may aspire.

In some communities in the Middle East and Southeast Asia, by contrast, polygyny is akin to a form of male conspicuous consumption, and a poor man in these communities would be considered rash for taking multiple wives.

Taking an additional wife might enable an educated man to reconcile the social imperative to respect group preferences regarding marriage (such as choosing a bride from his own village or ethnic group) with his individual preferences (such as for romantic fulfillment). Or it might enable a poor man to ensure his household's survival by maximizing its sources of food, labor and income. In any case, even in the absence of material rewards, possessing multiple wives is very often a marker of a man's social prestige, if not his greater wealth. A West African proverb holds that "A man with only one wife is the older brother of the bachelor"—in other words, his social standing is beneath that of men with multiple wives. Research in urban Mali and Senegal finds that the expectation of increased social status is among the factors motivating men's decisions to take additional wives. All else being equal, polygyny confers status advantages disproportionately on men.

Women, by contrast, have a very different status relationship with polygyny, particularly since they have less control than men over their entry into it. A woman may effectively choose polygynous status by agreeing to become the wife of an already-married man, but she may also find it thrust upon her when her husband takes another wife, oftentimes without her consent or even prior knowledge. Polygyny frequently goes hand in hand with kinship systems that require brides to leave their families (and often communities) of origin to integrate into new households and kin groups where they will have marginal status at best. Nowhere is polygyny (or, for that matter, polyandry) a privilege of elite women. In Africa, where it is most widespread, polygyny is positively correlated with women's rural residence, low educational attainment, and low socioeconomic status.

For this reason, a *single* woman may indeed stand to gain social standing through marriage to a polygynous husband, provided of course that he is economically successful. A *married* woman, however, generally sees the arrival of a co-wife as a threat (recall Barash's declaration that the arrival of a co-wife is "nearly always bad news" for the first wife). The newcomer is, from her perspective, a clear rival for the husband's time, affection, and resources; the newcomer's children will likewise be rivals of the first wife's children. To guard against such negative outcomes, in high-polygyny settings such as Senegal, wives in monogamous unions may accumulate savings outside their marital households, for example, by investing in land or housing. In doing so, they shore up their own futures and those of their children by preventing their own hard-earned income from benefiting prospective rivals, while also guarding against the potential of resource dilution that stems from sharing their husbands with co-wives. These motives may also explain why Senegalese women's rates of labor market participation rise in tandem with their risk of polygyny.

It is important to stress that female outlooks on polygyny are by no means uniformly negative. A woman may benefit from polygamous marriage in certain respects, particularly as she grows older. Her junior co-wife (or co-wives) may provide domestic help to ease her workload at home. She may well regard seeing less of her husband, and having sexual relations with him less often, as a desirable outcome; indeed, senior wives in some African societies experience a form of "social menopause" that is accompanied by higher social status and greater independence in their daily lives. In the highly patriarchal societies in which polygyny is most widespread, a woman in a polygynous marriage may claim the full social respect that comes with married status while gaining more autonomy over her own income and activities than enjoyed by her monogamously married peers. Such "benefits" may provide a senior wife modest relief from the strict gender norms and sex-segregated social structures that regulate her life. They are minor, however, compared to the social and economic rewards that a man stands to reap from his polygynous union.

THE DEMOGRAPHIC FOUNDATIONS OF POLYGYNOUS MARRIAGE MARKETS

The next thing we must grasp to better understand polygyny's various costs and benefits is the demography of plural marriage. People widely assume that when one husband marries an additional wife, he necessarily prevents a man from marrying altogether. Along with this assumption comes its corollary, that polygyny shuts men out of marriage and makes them losers in the Darwinian struggle to reproduce. We will explore some of these ideas' political implications in Chapter 5. Here, we will demonstrate how these assumptions diverge from polygyny's demographic realities.

Consider the case of Senegal, a majority-Muslim country in West Africa that is home to some of the highest polygyny rates on earth. At any given time, about a third of Senegalese husbands have more than one wife. If we assume a one-to-one ratio of polygynous husbands on one hand, and bachelors prevented from finding wives on the other, we would expect to see about a third of Senegalese men never marrying (and even that rate is only attainable if each polygynist marries just one additional wife). And yet, a 2017 survey showed that only *4 percent* of Senegalese men had never married by the time they reached their mid- to late-forties. Compare that to the United States, where more than 15 percent of men in the same age bracket had never married. Marriage, then, is all but universal in Senegal for men and women alike. In fact, despite their country's sky-high polygyny rate, Senegalese men enjoy better marriage odds than men in any Western country where polygyny is forbidden.

How is this possible? Could a large surplus of women exist in the Senegalese population? In fact, the assumption of a significant female surplus is widely held in high-polygyny societies. But this assumption also happens to be unfounded: Senegal has a relatively balanced sex ratio, with roughly 95 to 98 males per 100 females in the general population, and in this demographic aspect Senegal is typical of countries where polygyny rates are high. In all such countries, the male and female shares of the population are roughly even. Skewed sex ratios are not what allows widespread polygyny to coexist with near-universal marriage in this society.

Senegal's case is by no means unique: wherever we find high rates of polygyny, we almost always find universal or near-universal rates of marriage. Two demographic factors explain this coexistence. The first is high birth rates. Senegal has about 31 annual births per 1000 people in its population, and the average Senegalese woman in 2024 gave birth to about 4.2 children in her lifetime. The country's population has been growing by 2.5 to 3 percent annually, doubling roughly every three decades since the middle of the twentieth century. Figure 3.1 shows the distribution of Senegal's population by sex (horizontal axis) and age (vertical axis).

The second relevant demographic factor is the fact that men in high-polygyny societies tend to be significantly older than women

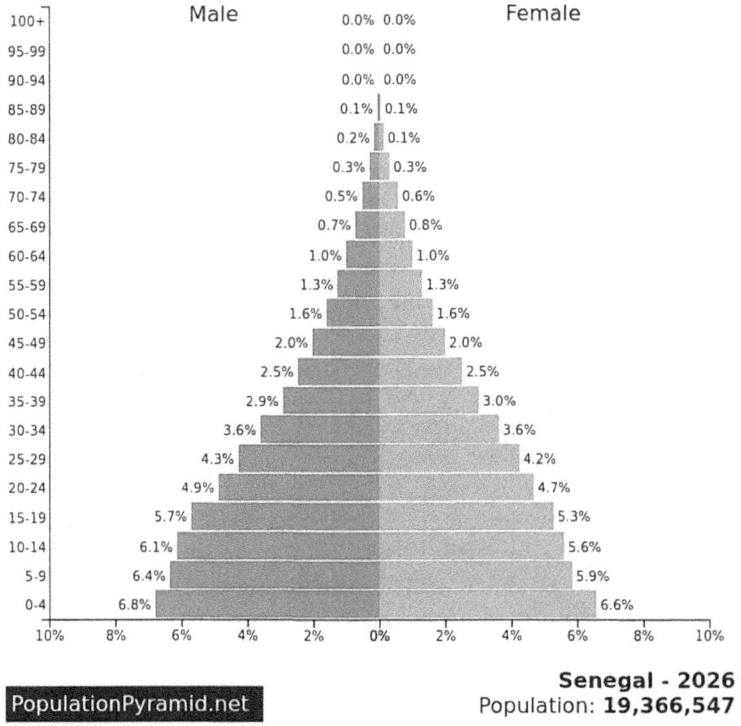

Figure 3.1 The age structure of Senegal's population, based on UN population data
Source: populationpyramid.net; https://www.populationpyramid.net/senegal/2026/

when they enter marriage. In Senegal, the mean age at first marriage is 20 years for females but 29 years for males. Such considerable age gaps are common in societies with high rates of polygyny. What explains these gaps? Studies have found consistent preferences among women for older mates and among men for younger mates in many societies, but this preference is by no means an innate human quality: in fact, it seems to diminish wherever gender equality increases. The age gap between spouses is not driven primarily by women's inclination to seek older mates; we must trace its origins elsewhere.

Now let us consider the marriage market, that process through which men and women are matched to one another through marriage. As noted earlier, this matching process is driven in some societies by senior kin and kin groups acting on behalf of brides and grooms; in other societies it is driven by brides and grooms themselves, often in concert with their parents or other relatives. The process is heavily influenced by the relative size of male and female cohorts entering the marriage market: when a male cohort is relatively smaller than its corresponding female cohort, for example, male cohort members enjoy more options and therefore more bargaining power in the matching process than female cohort members do. Such a sexual imbalance in a marriage market is called a "marriage squeeze."

To return to the Senegalese case, the nine-year gap between the mean male and female ages at first marriage, combined with demographic growth driven by high birth rates, yields *a marriage squeeze on women*. In Senegal in 2024, there were roughly 634,000 men between the ages of 30 and 34, and roughly 885,000 women between the ages of 20 and 24. In other words, there were about a third more women than men entering the Senegalese marriage market. Given these demographic facts, we might consider polygyny to be a "marriage market adjustment mechanism" enabling all entrants to the market to find a spouse. Men in Senegal are allowed to marry up to four wives, but most have just one, and only 20 percent of polygynous husbands ever have more than two wives at a time; in other words, Senegalese polygyny is what demographers call "low-intensity." This fact helps prevent a small number of highly successful (and mostly older) males from completely dominating the marriage market and monopolizing eligible brides.

The upshot is that while Senegalese men remain single longer (about nine years longer, on average) than Senegalese women do, nearly all of them *do* eventually marry. The country's high rate of polygyny does not shut men—even the less successful among them—out of the marriage market. In one sense, every male in Senegal is an "alpha." And Senegal's case fits the broader pattern in societies where polygyny is widespread: marriage rates are close to universal for men and women in these societies, and men are significantly older at first marriage than women are. We can summarize the relationship between demography and plural marriage by saying that high polygyny rates are generally driven not by sex imbalances in a population but by a system of gender norms and cultural structures that pushes women into early marriage and encourages them to remain married and to bear many children.

How does such a system work? Polygyny becomes truly prominent only in marriage markets where marriage-eligible women substantially outnumber marriage-eligible men—even when the overall population maintains a near-equal sex ratio. This demographic imbalance can arise through social and institutional mechanisms, as in Senegal or among Mormon fundamentalist communities, where practices such as the marginalization, delayed marriage, or expulsion of young men effectively reduce the pool of eligible males.

From the above discussion, it is clear that polygyny brings disproportionate benefits to older males, who make up the majority of polygynous husbands, and that these benefits come at the expense of younger males as well as females more generally. But this does not mean that polygyny *harms* younger males, at least not to the degree that many critics presume: young men in highly polygynous societies do not necessarily experience their delayed entry into marriage (relative to women's entry) as oppressive. Thanks to gendered double standards, they often face less social pressure than young women to marry young and to refrain from premarital sexuality.

REMARRIAGE AND POLYGYNY

To its traditionalist defenders, polygyny offers the benefit of making it easier for certain marginalized categories of women to participate in marriage markets. The first of these categories is widows. In some cultures, a widow is quickly married off to a brother of her deceased husband (a practice known as levirate marriage—see Chapter 1). From the Middle East to Mormon communities, widows have historically been among the most economically vulnerable women, a problem to which polygyny has often been offered as a solution. The Qur'an justifies polygyny in part through concern for widows; ten of the Prophet Muhammad's 11 wives were widows when he married them, including his first wife Khadijah. In some Islamic societies such as Bangladesh, widows rarely remarry, but in others (particularly in Africa) they are under strong pressure to remarry. In Senegal, during the 1980s, for example, a widow had a 91 percent chance of remarrying within five years of her husband's death, and upon remarriage faced a 75 percent chance of joining a polygynous marriage.

Divorcees constitute the other category of marginalized women for whom polygyny facilitates access to remarriage, and divorce is a major factor shaping highly polygynous marriage markets. As divorce has become more common and subject to less social stigma in many societies (part of a set of changes known as "the second demographic transition" that has swept much of the world since the late twentieth century), its significance in these markets has grown. The frequency of divorce varies considerably from one population to another, with rates as low as 10 percent and as high as 50 percent of all marriages. Divorce is a major component of all marriage systems where polygyny is widespread, and it works primarily in two ways: polygyny is often a leading cause of a woman's divorce, but divorce can also (via remarriage) lead to a woman's entry into a polygynous union. In West Africa, as we have seen, a woman who divorces her husband after he brings home a second wife frequently finds herself becoming the second wife of another man. In Burkina Faso, for example, 84 percent of women remarried within two years following divorce, and three-quarters of those within one year. Unsurprisingly, 69 percent of those divorcees eventually married into polygynous unions. And these remarriages may themselves be short-lived. In neighboring Benin during the 1980s, over 60 percent of marriages by men over age 50 ended in divorce. Divorce and remarriage are therefore common among women in the region, and for women remain a strategy for pursuing economic mobility. This pattern, moreover, extends far beyond the African continent: similar dynamics involving polygyny and divorce have been observed in Indonesia and Malaysia, for example.

In any society where plural marriage exists, then, widows and divorcees are indispensable for maintaining high levels of polygyny. Gendered cultural preferences, gender norms and taboos make single (and especially never-married) men in high-polygyny settings unlikely to wed widowed or divorced women, but those women can usually find polygynous husbands—a significant fact wherever cultural norms discourage women from living independently, as is the case in much of Africa and the Muslim world. Rather than treating "co-wife" as a fixed or definitive status, it is more accurate to recognize that in many cases it is temporary and often ends with divorce. Within Mormon fundamentalist communities, men seldom—if ever—divorce a wife. When marital relationships become too conflictual to resolve, husbands typically respond by taking an additional wife rather than dissolving existing unions. Women, by contrast, do initiate divorce and may either remarry or remain single. Most divorced women do remarry, and many find that men are readily willing to accept them as an additional co-wife (though, like their West African peers, these women are less likely to find monogamous husbands).

From both social and theological perspectives, men accrue higher spiritual or heavenly status by having three or more wives. Moreover, middle-aged women are rarely viewed as an economic burden, as they often bring independent sources of income into the household.

CONCLUSION

The benefits of polygyny are very much in the eye of the beholder. To some observers, polygyny offers the clear advantage of generating more offspring and higher social status—but these benefits go mainly to men rather than women. Polygyny also allows vulnerable categories of women to secure economic and social protection by remarrying into polygynous unions. These advantages too are relative, however, brought into being by patriarchal gender norms in societies where it is difficult or impossible for women to reside and earn their living independently of men. In some cases, particularly in communities where sisters might share a husband, cooperation between co-wives can provide significant labor savings to women. This benefit too is offset by cases of rivalry and competition, which appear frequently in the ethnographic record. The question of what polygyny's benefits are and who can collect them, therefore, can only be answered within the context of each particular culture and its associated values. We cannot define the benefits of any marriage practice without first determining what the purpose of marriage is, and that determination always depends on a culture-bound judgment.

FURTHER READING

Evolutionary psychologist David Barash's *Out of Eden: The Surprising Consequences of Polygamy* (2016) considers the lasting imprint of plural marriage on human biology and behavior. Barash argues that many contemporary social patterns, including male violence and the "battle of the sexes," are evolutionary leftovers from our species' polygynous past. His book examines how understanding these biological roots can help explain the challenges humans face in maintaining monogamous relationships today.

Economist Ester Boserup's *Woman's Role in Economic Development* (1970) pioneered the argument that polygyny arises in response to the needs of agricultural systems for women's labor. Her work highlights how modernization and colonial policies often undermined these traditional economic roles, frequently marginalizing women in the transition to industrial economies.

Miriam Koktvedgaard Zeitzen's anthropological study *Elite Malay Polygamy: Wives, Wealth and Woes in Malaysia* (2018) considers polygyny from the perspective of wealthy women in Malaysia's capital, Kuala Lumpur. While polygyny is relatively rare in this setting, the author contends that its presence creates significant emotional anxiety and social friction among elite urban dwellers.

BIBLIOGRAPHY

Barash, D. (2016). *Out of Eden: The surprising consequences of polygamy*. Oxford University Press.

Boserup, E. (1970). *Woman's role in economic development*. St. Martin's Press.

Koktvedgaard Zeitzen, M. (2018). *Elite Malay polygamy: Wives, wealth and woes in Malaysia*. Berghahn Books.

4

HOW DO THEY GET ALONG? POLYGYNOUS HOUSEHOLD DYNAMICS

LIVING ARRANGEMENTS

Residentially speaking, there are many ways to organize a polygynous marriage. We saw in Chapter 3 that in some cultures, most co-wives inhabit the same dwelling or compound, which enables them to collaborate in various chores, child rearing, and other household responsibilities. In other cultures, co-wives tend to reside in separate compounds, sometimes quite far apart, and may rarely even see one another. In some cultures, a polygynous husband may have no dwelling of his own and must spend each night in one of his wives' dwellings according to an agreed-upon schedule of turns. In other cultures, a husband either occupies a primary dwelling or has his own bedroom within a larger structure, in which his wives take turns spending the night.

Some scholars have sketched out an essential African model of polygyny in which the husband, all his wives and children reside together in the same compound. Among the Nyakyusa of Malawi or the Gusii of Kenya, for instance, each wife and her children occupied a separate and distinct segment of a residential compound. As represented by this African model, the entire polygynous household functions as a single unit for resource allocation, economic production, and the division of domestic labor. Wives may keep their earnings separate from the household budget within this arrangement, or they may contribute to a single common budget. Studies by Niara Sudarkasa and Obioma Nnaemeka highlight the egalitarian aspects of polygynous households

DOI: 10.4324/9781003628729-5

among the Yoruba of Nigeria, where they contend that the husband and his wives respect one another's prerogatives and positions within the unitary household structure.

As co-wives learn to work together and form alliances, the husband's authority becomes diffused, decentered, and often weakened. (As Paul Bohannan and Philip Curtin once put it, "If you think that one wife can henpeck a husband, you should see what three in league can do.") A semi-matrifocal arrangement may privately emerge that is quite advantageous to the wives in such a household; such matrifocal dynamics have sometimes been observed among polygynous Mormon families in the United States. According to Sudarkasa, friction is kept to a minimum—"if the women concerned respect each other's position within the household and if the man of the house shows no obvious preference for one [wife] over the other." As this chapter shows, however, these are two rather big ifs.

It would be wrong, moreover, to suppose either that a single "African model" of polygyny exists, or that polygyny is essentially egalitarian and cooperative, whether in Africa or anywhere else. The unitary, harmonious polygynous household described above is a common ideal type, but is by no means the norm. We have already seen that polygyny on the continent of Africa, whether in urban or rural settings, frequently leads to multilocal households in which there is little or no labor sharing among co-wives. The Kipsigi people in Kenya, for example, long preferred that a man's wives inhabit separate and distant homes specifically to minimize conflict.

Multilocal households are the dominant polygynous arrangement in Malaysia, where taking a new wife basically means establishing another household. If, in the coresidential ideal type championed by some of its advocates in Africa, polygyny *adds* labor and other resources to a man's household, multilocal models such as the one common in Malaysia *divide* husbands' resources among multiple distinct units made up of their wives and children. These contrasting models may help explain why polygyny has become an elite male privilege in Southeast Asia while remaining more generalized in Africa.

Stretching the multilocal household approach further, male rural-to-urban migrants in polygynous societies may live with one wife in the city while the other wife or wives remain in their community of origin, and the wives trade places at regular intervals (typically several months to a year). This is a common way to reduce the costs of plural marriage, as life in African or Asian villages tends to be much more affordable than in cities. By maintaining one or more wives in his rural community of origin, an absent migrant may also signal his continued membership in the community, retain rights to rural land, and provide care for his elderly parents. Indeed, parents may work to set their son up with a second wife in their village specifically to facilitate the latter outcome.

The multilocal model of polygyny stretches still further when men leave wives behind while they emigrate abroad. Among West African or Turkish migrants in the European Union, for instance, a man might marry a citizen of the host country to facilitate his legal status there while also maintaining one or more wives back home. In many such cases, these migrants' European wives are unaware of their co-wives' existence. "Transnational polygyny" can be extremely stressful for all parties involved. In the words of one scholar studying Senegalese migrants in France, as legal migration channels to France and other European countries have grown fewer and less accessible over time amid government crackdowns on immigration, migrants' transnational polygynous outcomes have become "less a premeditated strategy than an accommodation to an increasingly restrictive context."

DECISION-MAKING AND SENIORITY

In Niger, West Africa, writer Peter Chilson describes a polygamous family composed of a prominent local merchant and his four wives. The first wife ran a hotel the merchant owned some 300 miles away; the second wife ran a driving school he had helped her establish locally; the third and fourth wives were responsible for running the primary residence and its twenty-odd children, as well as managing the family's herd of livestock. "The marriage arrangement works like a small corporation," observes Chilson, "with a president (him) and four vice presidents." Their arrangement played to the strengths of each wife and allowed her to focus on the activities that mattered most to her.

Just as living space and residential arrangements shape a plural marriage, so does power. Power and responsibility may be apportioned within a polygynous household in very formal ways, as in the corporate structure Chilson encountered in Niger. While it is interesting to see how wives' roles may differ within such marriages, we should also remember that a polygynous husband almost always remains the primary decision-maker, while his wives have much less say over household affairs. In fact, as research in Burkina Faso has shown, wives in plural marriages might be less involved in family decision-making processes than wives in monogamous marriages living in the very same community.

There is much greater variability concerning relationships between co-wives. In many settings, rules of seniority regulate the prerogatives of each wife. These rules give a senior wife the right to assign domestic duties and apportion resources among her junior wives, settle disputes among wives, and often represent all the wives in discussions with their husband. She may therefore benefit from the labor of her juniors, receive more social respect, and command more influence within the household. Such rules of seniority exist in a broad range of cultures, from North America to northeastern India to the African continent. To cite a few West African examples: among Tombo fishing communities (Sierra Leone), a senior wife acts as the supervisor of the household's domestic labor; a senior wife in a Yoruba community (Nigeria), generally being past her child-bearing years, enjoys more opportunities than her juniors to conduct long-distance trade; in Balanta communities (Guinea-Bissau), a senior wife is responsible for recruiting her junior wives, whom she chooses among the girls of her own descent group, and whom she can send away at her pleasure.

Most often, a wife's seniority is based on the length of time she has spent in the marriage: the "first wife" is simply the one who has been married to the husband the longest. This is what confers seniority in most African cultures. Compared to African household organization, the fundamentalist Mormons are distinct. They do not rank wives by seniority but rather rely upon an ad hoc and unvoiced informal hierarchy based on the husband's preference. The fundamentalist preference for flexibility can enable an incoming or junior wife to become the husband's favorite wife (discussed below), especially if the first wife's marriage remained cold, distant, and hostile. In the African case the story is different. In this system a junior wife's advancement occurs when a senior wife dies or leaves the marriage, or when the husband takes a newer, more junior wife who will be ranked below all the other wives.

The possibility of advancement in seniority means that polygyny becomes more appealing to a woman as she advances through the life course. In Sierra Leone, notes anthropologist Caroline Bledsoe, young women are typically wary of polygyny and the demands of senior wives, but "as they grow older and gain junior wives of their own, their opinions of polygyny often improve." A post-menopausal woman enjoying seniority has earned the recognition of her peers and juniors, greater influence within the family, and more control over how she spends her time.

Sometimes rank accrues by means other than time spent within marriage. For example, in certain Bamiléké communities of Cameroon, the senior co-wife is elected by all the women of the household. In contexts of sororal polygyny, such as among the Achuar of Ecuador or the Mardudjara of Australia, a wife has seniority because she is the older sister, not necessarily because she entered the marriage first (although a younger sister is unlikely to marry before any of her older sisters).

Seniority is not always an asset for a wife in a polygynous marriage. It sometimes degrades her actual status and privileges within the household. In polygynous Israeli Bedouin families, for instance, husbands typically favor their younger wives, leading to senior wives' material and emotional neglect. There are also contexts in which seniority is irrelevant, such as among the Yakö (Nigeria) or elite families in Kuala Lumpur (Malaysia), where no hierarchy among co-wives is possible because there are no co-wife relations to begin with. Finally, various factors can undermine a wife's seniority. In a pro-natalist African context, for example, a childless first wife may command little to no authority over her junior wives who have borne children. In an Egyptian Bedouin context, a junior wife who belongs to the same paternal lineage as her husband may enjoy better treatment from him than a senior wife who belongs to a different lineage. In a highly status-conscious social context, a first wife from a low-status family may be treated as inferior to her junior co-wife from a higher-ranking family. Finally, *how* a wife got married—through a formal or informal ceremony, a civil wedding or religious ritual—can affect her standing, bargaining power, and influence within the household. Any or all these factors can upset the official ranking among wives.

And then there are the problems that arise when husbands play favorites.

EQUITY VERSUS FAVORITISM

Favoritism is without a doubt the thorniest issue affecting the practice of polygyny. From Saudi Arabia to Suriname, women's most common complaints about their polygynous unions concern their husbands' lack of fairness toward them. In many cultures, a host of cultural norms and religious injunctions requires polygynous husbands to treat their wives equitably. But enacting equity within one's plural marriage and having it accepted as such by all spouses is much more easily said than done.

A big part of the problem is that however much they feel obliged to show the same love and favor toward each of their wives, polygynous husbands cannot help but develop favorites among them. Even in cultures where religious law and social norms require equitable treatment among co-wives, common terms exist to designate the preferred wife. In Senegal, for example, people know well that when an elderly man takes a younger woman as his "retirement wife," he will likely treat her as his favorite.

A man's favorite is not always the youngest wife, the most senior wife, or the most attractive wife, but she is someone with whom he shares a special, intimate relationship that he does not or cannot replicate with any of her co-wives. Although fundamentalist Mormon leaders warn constantly against developing emotionally exclusive bonds in a polygynous marriage, their followers widely recognize that such bonds are difficult to avoid. Similarly, people in Muslim communities *understand* that Islamic law expressly forbids a husband from showing any special treatment toward one of his wives, yet it is difficult to find co-wives who do not perceive some degree of favoritism in their husband's marital conduct. Islam's holiest book, the Qur'an, offers little comfort in this regard, advising men: "Howsoever you may try, you will never be able to treat your wives equally" (sura 4, verse 129). Still, men endeavor to keep up the appearance of equal treatment and equal affection.

The resources and time that a husband devotes to each of his wives can, in many cases, be quantified and compared. Yet even when these turn out to be evenly distributed, and sleeping rosters carefully adhered to, and all spouses have made a conscientious effort to follow the rules, a husband can still develop a stronger emotional attachment to one of his wives, and it will be difficult for him to prevent the other wives from discerning his favoritism.

In the absence of overt favoritism, polygynous husbands frequently struggle to determine what constitutes equitable treatment of their wives. Suppose a man has one wife with three children who doesn't work outside the home, and another wife with no children who does. Would it be fair if he made identical monetary contributions to each wife, or should he treat each according to her unique situation? If he took one wife on a private vacation, must he then treat his other wives to the same vacation in turn, even if they don't care for the destination? Community norms often prescribe solutions in such cases, but at the heart of this problem is the fact that each human being has different preferences and endowments, ensuring that there is no entirely objective way to determine what constitutes equitable treatment toward any two of them.

Moreover, co-wives are unlikely to wait passively to see which of them their husband takes a special liking to. Instead, they mobilize their own economic, social, and sexual resources to curry favor with him. In a monogamous household where the risk of polygyny is high, a woman might do everything in her power to prevent her husband from taking another wife. If she fails in this regard, she may be willing to pay a high price to become his favorite spouse. Thus, many co-wives are pitted against each other in unrelenting competition. Even a senior wife may find the advantages of her seniority greatly reduced, if not eliminated altogether, by this rivalry. This rivalry will be discussed later.

Husbands profit very deliberately from the competitive dynamic within their polygynous households. In fact, a man may decide to bring another wife into his home expressly to check his first wife's power; to quote a Moroccan saying reported by sociologist Fatima Mernissi, "Debase a woman by bringing in another one." The husband, having established his polygynous household, exploits the atmosphere of tension fueled by this competition and plays his wives off against one another in a classic divide-and-rule maneuver. Interviews with polygynous husbands in Mali reveal the comfort that men take from this strategy. In the words of one interviewee, "If you enjoy peace twenty percent of the time as a monogamous husband, once you marry a second wife you have peace sixty percent of the time. It multiplies your happiness." In high-polygyny communities, men increasingly hear such accounts from their peers as they get older. Even if they began their married lives as committed monogamists, men become ever more likely to seek plural unions as they approach middle age to pursue higher status, greater marital control, or some combination of both.

DIVISION OF RESOURCES

Resources can be distributed within the polygynous household in many ways, which vary by culture and economic activity. In agricultural settings where polygyny is common, a man may allocate his family's harvest as a single unit for his wives to ration and prepare collectively for the entire household. Alternatively, he may divide the harvest among his wives, whether equally or differentially according to the number of children living with each wife. But while this household-level division of resources applies to the family's common harvest, wives may also have production from their own individual plots, and sometimes other sources of private income.

Quite frequently, wives in polygynous marriages maintain more control over these private resources than their peers in monogamous marriages. While they must contribute their labor to serve the needs of the entire household, and while they have less participation in household decisions, polygynous wives do tend to have greater control over their own earnings. They often maintain separate budgets from those of their co-wives and husbands, enabling them to accumulate resources over which their husbands have no legitimate claim. A degree of economic autonomy is among the greatest benefits of polygyny to women, at least in many African communities.

CO-WIFE COOPERATION

Before turning to the problems that arise between wives, let's examine the prospects for them to work together. These prospects appear to be greatest in cases of sororal polygyny, as the sisterly bond generally promotes partnership and harmony among co-wives. According to a Zulu saying, "The love of two sisters overcomes the jealousy of polygyny." Indeed, from Australia to South Africa, sororal polygyny seems to correlate well with co-wife cooperation.

As mentioned above, women in many polygynous contexts dread the prospect of having to share their husbands with other wives, and they do whatever they can to prevent polygyny in their household; nevertheless, their husbands may bring home additional wives without consulting or even informing their existing wives. In other contexts, however, women participate actively in choosing their husbands' new wives and may even prevent their husbands from making the selection on their own. Some women claim to be eager to have co-wives and may press their husbands to take additional wives. This pattern has been observed both in sororal and non-sororal polygynous communities. Where marriage is understood and experienced more as an economic arrangement than an exclusive intimate relationship, where labor power is crucial for a household's economic success, and where co-wives live together, such a preference on a wife's part makes practical sense. A new co-wife can help with household chores and childcare, with farm labor, or with income-generating activities. In a Talen village in Ghana, anthropologist Meyer Fortes observed that women in polygynous households showed great voluntary mutual support for their co-wives and didn't object to their husbands bringing new wives into the household. Some even came to refer to their co-wives as their sisters.

In other cases, women in a polygynous marriage follow a more instrumental approach toward forging relationships with their co-wives. An African-American Muslim woman interviewed by Debra Majeed, for example, said that she got involved in the selection of her new co-wife as a form of "emotional insurance" against subsequent domestic conflict, and felt that her participation made it easier for the two of them to start their relationship off on a friendly footing. Co-wives often maintain respectful distance from one another and collaborate pragmatically when circumstances allow. Rigid control by male household heads and senior wives can facilitate efficient if not eager cooperation among wives, and maintaining a wide interval between the ages of wives in a household can even foster friendship in some cases.

Finally, co-wives sometimes join forces to influence or force a husband to change his behavior. A neglectful husband, for example, may find himself facing the united opposition of his wives. Among Mormon fundamentalists this was a constant anxiety, but it seems to have never occurred as each wife pursued her own interest independent of the other wives. The few times co-wives did unite was when they attacked a junior incoming wife. Many a polygynous husband does his best to avoid this outcome by playing his wives against each other, making them less likely to recognize shared grievances or find common cause.

Some scholars have highlighted the room for goodwill and cooperation within polygynous households. While acknowledging the existence of some rivalry, for instance, Niara Sudarkasa described the relationships among the co-wives of a Yoruba residential compound as "characterized by a considerable degree of camaraderie and cooperation." Such positive dynamics appear to be outliers in the ethnographic record, however. As we have seen, many women prefer to live separately from their co-wives, thus forfeiting any of the domestic advantages that might come from a close relationship with them. More significantly, a large body of research across cultures shows rivalry among co-wives to be a pervasive and significant problem.

COMPETITION AND CONFLICT

Paul Bohannan and Philip Curtin point out that "in many African languages, the word for co-wife springs from the same root as the word for jealousy." This close association between polygyny and rivalry is by no means limited to societies on the African continent. In South America, among the Saramaka people of Suriname, a synonym of the verb "to fight" is "to act like a co-wife," as arguments and even physical altercations are not unusual between a man's wives.

A cross-cultural survey of 39 African and 30 non-African cultural groups practicing non-sororal polygyny sorted these groups into four categories based on relations among co-wives: (1) those in which conflict was endemic, (2) those characterized by pragmatic cooperation punctuated by intense conflict, (3) those characterized by pragmatic cooperation with occasional hostility, and

(4) those in which relations were harmonious. The survey found co-wife hostility to be present, at least to some degree, in all 69 groups; none was classified as harmonious. Conflict was present regardless of a group's system of kinship or mode of subsistence.

Rivalry therefore appears to be a structural element of non-sororal polygynous marriage. Comparing polygynous households to monogamous ones, economists' field research has found polygynists less efficient and cooperative (based on experimental cooperation games in western Nigeria) while also more prone to anxiety, disputes, and intimate partner violence (based on randomized control trials of cash transfers in Mali). Disputes arise over a wide range of issues, but here we will focus on co-wife competition in two key areas.

First is the problem of favoritism discussed above. Whether with respect to sexual access, food and living allowances, or gifts, polygynous husbands are susceptible to showing partiality and their wives are prone to see evidence of partiality. Research in Senegal has found that even if a husband himself is scrupulously fair toward his wives, each of them is incentivized by her need for social status and psychological ease to claim the status of favored wife, convincing her co-wives that the husband takes better care of her. His own relatives may also seek to sow perceptions of unfair treatment among his wives so as to divide them against one another. As mentioned above, since no two wives are the same in personality or preference, it is never simple to determine what constitutes equitable treatment of them; savvy individuals exploit this ambiguity for their own purposes.

Children constitute another major area of conflict. In strongly pronatalist cultures, whether in Africa or in fundamentalist Mormon communities, co-wives compete over who can bear the most children, often under the impression that reproductive success is the surest way to retain the husband's affection and support. This competitive fertility then leads to competitive child rearing, with each wife determined that her children be recognized as the most cherished or accomplished. Rivalries thus erupt over children's access to schooling, their school performance, and later over their economic achievements, especially for sons. In one Senegalese community where having emigrant sons is a sign of social status, co-wives compete over whose son will be the first to establish himself abroad, and each pressures her sons accordingly. As they get older, the children growing up in polygynous households compete for their father's attention and regard. Competition among half-siblings is a fundamental social dynamic of many African societies, where it is seen as a driving force behind innovation and progressive social change, celebrated in oral epics and the lyrics of popular songs.

There are sinister sides to these rivalries, however (see Chapter 2). Whether among co-wives or their children, competition often leads to threats and violence. A woman might seek to poison her co-wife or her children or use sorcery against them in her bid to vanquish her and her children's rivals. The fear of such dangers is ever-present in many polygynous households in West Africa, and the costs add up in numerous ways.

Despite this grim picture, however, it would be wrong to suggest that polygyny inevitably leads to disputes, violence, and ill health. Some communities and families have managed to mitigate the risks discussed above.

HIGH-FUNCTIONING POLYGYNOUS FAMILIES

After surveying hundreds of Bedouin families in Israel's Negev Desert, social workers Alean Al-Krenawi and Verem Slonim-Nevo categorized the polygynous families in their sample into two types: "high-functioning" and "low-functioning." Husbands in high-functioning families had the same motives for entering polygyny as husbands in low-functioning families, namely the desire for social status, more sons, and in some cases greater control in their households. Beyond this measure, however, there were many divergences. By their own accounts, husbands in high-functioning families sought their first wives' permission before bringing home additional wives, while husbands in low-functioning families simply brought new wives home without consulting their existing wives. In interviews, husbands in high-functioning families spoke frequently about the need to respect their wives, while husbands in low-functioning families did not. Husbands in high-functioning families spent more time with their children and knew more details about their children's lives, while husbands in low-functioning families were more distant from their children. Wives in high-functioning families were calm and accepting, and recognized the authority of senior wives, while wives in low-functioning families were hostile toward each other and did not recognize seniority. Finally, children in high-functioning families had warm relations with their parents and siblings, while children in low-functioning families tended to be estranged.

After reading this breakdown, one might object that by erecting their two opposing categories, these researchers created their own definition of *what* constitutes "high" and "low" functioning in polygynous households without explaining *why* some of these families work together harmoniously while others do not. In this regard, scholarly research in a diversity of settings offers a few potential "best practices" for high-functioning polygyny. These include time-honored examples that could apply to any marriage or even any relationship, such as maintaining open communication, fair treatment, and mutual respect.

Some recommendations, though, are specific to polygyny. Perhaps the most common is that co-wives should not live together. Almost everywhere polygyny is practiced, observers have found that cohabitation entails too much friction and potential for conflict. High-functioning families tend to be those in which co-wives maintain spatial separation without being completely removed from one another's lives. But separation brings with it another challenge: how can co-wives verify that their husband is treating them equitably if they do not see each other regularly? To minimize suspicions of favoritism, polygynous husbands whose wives live separately must take extra steps to ensure accountability and transparency in how they deal with their dependents. Some polygynous communities, such as the fundamentalist Mormons studied by Jankowiak, continue to hold up shared residence as an ideal, but these groups are in a shrinking minority.

Another recommendation is to maintain clear systems of household organization and authority; where these are absent, families are at greater risk of breaking down. Such systems might include procedures for integrating a new wife into the household (cited as a hallmark of high-functioning polygynous Mormon families). Bambara farmers in Mali have practiced a kind of marital apprenticeship by which senior wives trained new wives to negotiate the transition into their households. High-functioning households have also developed some procedures to reduce friction between co-wives and their children. Among the most common of these is the practice in which co-wives raise each other's children; this practice of intra-household child fostering has been documented among fundamentalist Mormons and West Africans alike. In the West African context, it helps that child fostering, whether short- or long-term, is a longstanding institution in many cultures: up to a third of children in different parts of the region typically live apart from their biological parents at any given time.

There is evidence, however, that customary practices for regulating polygyny and preventing conflict within polygynous households are in decline, particularly in Africa. The institution of wife seniority has been undermined by the growing influence of Islam, which emphasizes equality among co-wives. Intra-household child fostering practices too are being abandoned in many settings. In The Gambia and Mali, for example, while adults interviewed during the 2010s were aware of such practices and some of them had been fostered as children by their mothers' co-wives, none currently lived in households where co-wives were raising each other's children. In these and other cultural contexts, polygynists themselves increasingly regard such customs as incompatible with mothers' rights over their own children, and with modern life more generally. It has never been easy to achieve high-functioning polygyny, but as traditional safeguards against domestic conflict fall away, the state of harmony within a polygynous family will likely become even more difficult to accomplish.

CONCLUSION: THE FUTURE OF POLYGYNOUS ARRANGEMENTS

It should be evident by now that there are few universal truths about polygynous households, the rules by which they live, the extent to which their members get along with each other, or whether such households are cooperative or conflict-ridden. One reason for this difficulty is the fact that polygyny is always practiced in specific cultural contexts, the influence of which is significant over household- and individual-level outcomes. For example, in a West African community where many children are fostered out to other relatives or to non-relatives, the idea that co-wives would raise each other's children might not strike many people as unusual or objectionable, and most children growing up in such a system would not perceive themselves as having been deprived of a nurturing, positive upbringing, nor even to have lived abnormal childhoods. In other cultural settings, however, this same idea would be a non-starter, widely considered a violation of the "natural bonds" between mothers and their biological children.

Two conclusions that we can comfortably reach are that conflict is inevitable in polygynous households, and that some degree of rivalry or competition infuses relations between the wives of the same husband. A vast body of social research from around the world confirms these conclusions. Beyond these safe generalizations, however, there is great variation. Some polygynous marriages work better than others when they have specific practices for minimizing inter-wife rivalries and promoting husbands' equitable treatment of wives. These practices are not replicable everywhere, and even where they have been established for generations, some appear to be fading away.

The growing preference for a man's wives to be housed separately is one trend that has transformed polygynous household dynamics in many parts of the world and that seems likely to continue. This trend might be accompanied by lower levels of conflict among co-wives, and perhaps also by lower prevalence of the psychological, medical, and social stressors that scholars have so often observed in polygynous families (see Chapter 2). But it will also reshape families in high-polygyny communities, perhaps contributing to the dissolution of extended families that historically have brought together full- and half-siblings into a single domestic structure. If the children of future polygynists may therefore be freed of certain burdens by this reconfiguration of polygynous living arrangements, they will also live in fundamentally different kinship worlds marked by little contact with their fathers' other wives or their children. Polygynists' wives and offspring may face lower risk of domestic conflict in this emerging future, but they will also have fewer means at their disposal to curb conflicts that do break out.

FURTHER READING

African Systems of Kinship and Marriage, edited by A. R. Radcliffe-Brown and Daryll Forde (1950), is a classic anthropological collection, many chapters of which highlight the significance of polygyny in African cultures. Niara Sudarkasa's *Where Women Work: A Study of Yoruba Women in the Marketplace and in the Home* (1973) is an ethnographic case study of women and marriage in a West African community where polygyny is widespread. Mariama Ba's novel *So Long a Letter* (originally published in French as *Une Si Longue Lettre* in 1979) recounts the travails of a married Senegalese mother whose husband takes a second wife.

BIBLIOGRAPHY

Ba, M. (1981). *So long a letter* (M. V. De Jager, Trans.). Heinemann. (Original work published 1979.)

Radcliffe-Brown, A. R., and Forde, D. (Eds.). (1950). *African systems of kinship and marriage*. Oxford University Press.

Sudarkasa, N. (1973). *Where women work: A study of Yoruba women in the marketplace and in the home*. University of Michigan Press.

5

POLYGYNY AND INEQUALITY

POLYGYNY AT THE MACRO LEVEL

In Chapters 3 and 4, we have considered polygyny at the micro level, centering on the question of whose lives most benefit from it and whose are most harmed by it, as well as the question of how polygynous households function. But what effects might polygyny have *above* the level of individuals and households? This chapter expands our focus to consider the ways that polygyny can shape large human populations, those of entire nations and even civilizations. In particular, we examine a subject that has long fascinated scholars: the relationship between polygyny and social inequality. Many scholars believe that polygyny is inextricably tied to forms of inequality that fuel societal tensions and violence; in light of this association, some have proposed that polygyny be banned.

Before we can turn to those subjects, however, we first need to review theories about why polygynous forms of marriage, once widespread around the world, lost ground to monogamous ones. These theories are helpful for thinking about the effects polygyny can have on human societies, especially where inequality is concerned.

WHY DID MONOGAMY BECOME DOMINANT? FIVE THEORIES

As noted in Chapter 1, a long historical perspective shows that polygyny has been practiced in the vast majority of recorded human cultures—roughly 84 percent, in fact. Yet a global trend

DOI: 10.4324/9781003628729-6

away from polygyny seems to have taken hold over the past few centuries, with monogamous marriage becoming the only officially accepted form of marriage in a growing number of societies. This monogamous trend spread very gradually at first, expanding from western Europe to envelop most of North and South America and much of Asia. By the twenty-first century, at least two-thirds of all countries had outlawed plural marriage. Even in African and Middle Eastern countries where polygyny remains lawful, and where polygyny rates are still high relative to other world regions, the practice of polygyny over the past few decades has tended to decline. Observing this trend, many scholars have asked, "Why monogamy? What accounts for the success of the monogamous marriage model?"

One theory revolves around male inequality and female choice. This is related to the female choice model encountered in Chapter 3 that explains polygyny as the product of women choosing male partners with the most resources. When a society's resources are limited, it usually results in stark inequalities that enhance a successful man's mate attractiveness as a viable spouse capable of supporting his wives and their children. By this reasoning, when resource inequality is high among men (in other words, when there is a wide disparity of wealth), polygyny too will be high. Conversely, the female choice model suggests that when differences in wealth among male suitors are low, women are more likely to opt for monogamous unions. This explanation is problematic, however, given that monogamy came to be normative in many societies where levels of socioeconomic inequality were surging amid the economic transformations of the early modern era. Doubts also persist that women would have had much freedom to choose their partners or to resist marriages they didn't want in these societies, many of which remain highly patriarchal and limit the autonomy of young unmarried people, particularly females (see Chapter 1).

Another theory suggests that as a society becomes more specialized and its division of labor more pronounced, its high-status men strategize to limit or eliminate polygyny in order to retain the political support of low-status men. This "male compromise theory" thus sees monogamy coming to social prominence as a result of an elite bargain, struck initially in medieval Europe and later spreading to other world regions, intended to facilitate access to the marriage market for the masses of poor men and thereby to head off the destabilizing political effects of too many men finding themselves unable to marry and reproduce. While male compromise theory is logically plausible, historical evidence that elites ever deliberately chose such a bargain is lacking. A more recent version of this theory suggests that as levels of male wealth rose in society, women gained latitude to exercise their preference for monogamy, even if sometimes in the form of "serial monogamy"—that is, elite men marrying and divorcing multiple women in succession.

According to a third theory, monogamy came to dominate because social transformations altered parental investment strategies. Under the old agrarian order in which polygyny was more common, fathers were incentivized to raise more children and to invest less (especially in terms of education) in each child. Having more wives, irrespective of the quality of each wife and her level of human capital, was advantageous under these conditions. As societies moved toward industrial production and human capital became more important to economic survival, fathers were incentivized to raise fewer children and to make greater investments in each. A man came to value a wife's quality more highly if she could contribute to those investments in their children. This theory focuses on the sources as well as the level of male inequality in a society, and predicts that as returns on human capital investments increase in a modernizing economy, monogamy will also tend to increase.

The fourth theory we consider here pertains to group competition. This theory shares a key assumption of some of the previous theories, namely that high levels of polygyny are inherently disruptive to society because they exacerbate male sexual competition that leaves too many men unable to marry. To quote evolutionary psychologist David Buss, "The more polygynous the culture, the more some men will be inclined to pursue high-risk tactics in an effort to gain status, resources, and mates." In small-scale societies, this dynamic can lead to conflict as men seek to capture women from other groups. In large-scale societies, it has been linked to higher risk of civil war. By contrast, higher levels of monogamy tend to "level the reproductive playing field," promoting greater social cohesion by reducing crime and conflict. Monogamy also encourages parental investment in children, leading to greater economic productivity and savings. A trio of scholars led by Joseph Henrich offered a related cultural historical explanation for the rise of monogamy in western Europe, arguing that it was the authority of the Catholic Church to assert its morality into the lives of commoners and the aristocracy who, whatever their personal feelings, were restricted to marriage to one person. The new theological ideal highlighted monogamous marriage as the only allowable and thus viable institution for cultural transmission of decent rights. By this theory, groups that adopt monogamous marriage norms will out-compete groups that do not, and will be more likely to flourish over the long run.

The final theory we consider pertains to the relationship between polygyny and disease. Biologist Bobbi Low predicted that in human populations with high levels of "pathogen stress" (elevated prevalence of pathogens leading to a heavy burden of disease), a woman would be more likely to choose polygyny with a "high quality" male over monogamy with a low-quality male in order to ensure the greatest odds of survival for her offspring. She therefore hypothesized that rates of polygyny would be positively correlated with pathogen stress. Comparing data from an ethnographic atlas to the distribution of seven infectious diseases (including malaria and leprosy), Low found an association between the presence of these diseases and the rate of polygynous marriage in a society. She reasoned that in settings of high pathogen stress, women chose to enter polygyny under the assumption that a polygynous husband would be a good provider and contribute to their children's increased resistance to disease. She likewise reasoned that men used polygyny to increase their offspring's genetic variation and with it their disease resistance.

While all of these theories can add to our understanding of the global trend toward monogamy, none has gained a dominant position in the bid to explain monogamy's historical ascendancy. As we will see, however, they have collectively shaped scholars' understandings of polygyny's impact on societies today. In the sections below, we examine related arguments about the relationship between polygyny and inequality, underdevelopment, and conflict in contemporary countries.

DOES POLYGYNY MAKE COUNTRIES POORER?

In the early 2000s, economist Michèle Tertilt analyzed marriage data, birthrates, and economic productivity data in a set of tropical countries. She discerned a pattern: those countries where polygyny was legal and widespread (mostly in sub-Saharan Africa) diverged demographically and economically from countries where polygyny was illegal. The average age gap between spouses was much higher (6.4 years) in the polygynous countries than in the monogamous ones (2.8 years). The birthrate was 6.78 children per woman in the polygynous countries, compared to 4.62 in the monogamous ones. Investment rates and capital-output ratios were significantly lower in polygynous countries. Poverty was also highest in high-polygyny African countries, with per capita Gross Domestic Product (GDP) 38 percent lower than in low-polygyny African countries.

Tertilt developed a model incorporating marriage patterns, birthrates, and savings to study these differences. In her model, polygyny drove up birthrates and concentrated a significant portion of household spending on children. She predicted that the legal abolition of polygyny in high-polygyny countries would lower their birthrates by 40 percent, increase savings by 70 percent, and raise per capita economic output by 170 percent. While she recognized that polygyny was not the sole cause of poverty, she concluded that it "might be an important contributing factor to the continuing underdevelopment of sub-Saharan Africa." She speculated that this problem could be addressed by some type of "enforced monogamy."

How might polygyny contribute to poverty? Tertilt reasoned that it does so by inflating demand for wives, which in turn drives up bridewealth payments. Men's higher spending on getting married crowds out investment in "alternative assets." Under these conditions, spending on acquiring wives takes precedence over investing in economically productive capital.

Like all models, Tertilt's model simplifies highly complex social processes by focusing on a few variables while excluding others. It also makes some dubious assumptions: it posits that an average spousal age gap in polygamous societies is around 15 years (it is typically five to ten), and presumes that a legal ban would effectively change behavior in high-polygyny countries. Nevertheless, her model demonstrates some of the mechanisms through which the practice of polygyny might affect society at large, and has therefore proven quite influential.

A pair of economists, David de la Croix and Fabio Mariani, subsequently developed their own model of the relationship between polygyny and poverty that looked at this relationship from a different perspective. They considered how a society's distribution of wealth might affect its institutions of marriage. Their model, based on a political-economic framework rather than empirical data from specific countries, posits that a low number of wealthy individuals in a society will tend to perpetuate polygyny by favoring a marital alliance between rich men and poor women. As the level of wealth in a society increases and the number of rich men grows, they predicted, more women would be able to marry wealthy men without having to share their husbands with other wives. As women shifted toward monogamous unions, prospects for their children's social mobility would rise as monogamous husbands would invest more in their children's human capital. This dynamic would then create a feedback loop: a society with growing numbers of wealthy men marrying monogamously would tend to see greater economic prospects for its offspring, and greater economic growth in the long term. By contrast, a society mired in poverty would discourage monogamous norms from taking root, diminish investments in human capital, and ultimately fail to develop the social and economic institutions leading to the creation of wealth. Under the assumptions of de la Croix and Mariani's model, then, the conditions of poverty—in particular, the shortage of wealthy men—make it more difficult for a society to transition to monogamy. Polygyny may not keep countries poor, by this reasoning, but poverty seems to keep many countries polygynous.

DOES POLYGYNY MAKE COUNTRIES MORE VIOLENT?

In the early years of the twenty-first century, data from African demographic surveys revealed a curious finding: women in high-polygyny societies were more likely to justify intimate partner violence against women than women in low-polygyny societies. Overall, female respondents in these surveys were twice as likely as male respondents to make statements justifying women's domestic abuse. These and similar findings have served to illuminate larger-scale political violence in many societies where polygyny is prevalent.

Informed by evolutionary theory, psychologist Satoshi Kanazawa used ethnographic and conflict-related academic datasets to search for a statistical correlation between polygyny and warfare. He posited that polygynous marriage systems deprive large numbers of men from marriage and reproduction, and he hypothesized that the frustrated ambitions of these surplus men would fuel civil war. From his analysis of the data, Kanazawa concluded that polygyny is the "first law of intergroup conflict"—in other words, the prevalence of polygyny in a country is a strong predictor of that country's likelihood of experiencing a civil war.

Other scholars, informed by feminist theory, have tried to highlight the mechanisms that brutalize women, destabilize societies and states, and generate large-scale conflict. Inequality and polygyny have featured prominently in all these analyses. Rose McDermott, in the book *The Evils of Polygyny*, has drawn a direct line from polygynous marriage to violence, using a much broader set of empirical statistics than Tertilt or other researchers had available to them. Analyzing data from the WomenStats database of 171 countries, McDermott and colleagues found polygyny globally to be associated with social harm—i.e., positively correlated with ill health, lower life expectancy, violence against women and children, crime, political instability, and warfare. Just as troubling, they found no correlations between polygyny and any positive social outcomes.

McDermott came to the conclusion that the correlations with social harm must stem from the same logical process evoked by previous theories about polygyny and inequality: when some men take multiple wives, sex ratios (at least in the marriage market) are skewed by the presence of "surplus males" unable to find wives. "Many men, often a majority, have no wives at all in societies where polygyny is prevalent," she writes. "This imbalance is the crux of what precipitates widespread societal effects of violence based on individual patterns of sexual behavior." Frustrated by their inability to marry and lacking any social safety net from their impoverished governments, these surplus males are ripe for recruitment by criminal gangs, political extremists, religious radicals, and terrorist groups. In this manner, writes McDermott, "polygyny for the few" brings about "mass dislocation and violence for the majority" in society.

In light of this analysis, McDermott argues that polygyny fuels many of the problems faced by people living in unstable countries, particularly women and girls. Conventional efforts to empower females through education, labor force participation and political representation, she added, would not suffice to relieve the burden of violence and gender subjugation as long as they failed to confront the problem of polygyny.

In their book *The First Political Order*, political scientists Valerie Hudson, Donna Bowen, and Perpetua Nielsen undertake a similar analysis of the sources of social discord and political violence using the WomenStats database. Whereas McDermott focuses on polygyny alone as the linchpin of unjust social orders, Hudson and colleagues pursue a broader approach. They identify a set of social practices, which they label the "Patriarchal/Fraternal Syndrome," that boost inequality, subordinate women, and exacerbate conflict in many unstable countries. This syndrome is a system of control that starts at the level of household organization and expands to weaken the nation-state itself. In addition to polygyny, the authors list ten practices constituting this syndrome: violence against women, patrilocal marriage, early marriage, legal discrimination, restrictions on women owning property, bridewealth and dowry, son preference and sex ratio alteration, cousin marriage, impunity for the killing of women, and the treatment of rape as a property crime against men.

In naming the Patriarchal/Fraternal Syndrome and enumerating its components, Hudson and colleagues sought to expose the interlocking social and cultural institutions that act in concert to constrain women and perpetuate unjust social orders. The discrimination, authoritarianism, and violence of states in many countries, they argue, are simply a scaled-up version of the same social forces that keep females subordinated in their families and marriages. The male-controlled patrilineal kin groups or clans that constrain women and girls' marital options and that threaten women and girls with violence in the home have become embedded in these country's governing structures, creating dysfunctional states characterized by corruption, instability, and conflict.

While polygyny is just one component of the Patriarchal/Fraternal Syndrome, Hudson and colleagues contend, it plays quite an important role. Elite males acquire multiple wives to signal their high status and to broker marriage alliances with other elite males. In rural agrarian settings, polygynous marital arrangements also make it easier for male household heads to command labor and accumulate wealth. Meanwhile, these men's financial expenses for acquiring new wives leaves less capital for investing in the health, education, and nutrition of their households' wives and children. Polygyny additionally drives up bridewealth, a major obstacle to young men's marriage prospects. But the primary problem of polygyny, according to Hudson and her coauthors, is that it "produces especially unstable societies, because it means that certain men in the clan will have several mates, whereas others may have none, undermining the solidarity necessary among the men of the group." Marriage markets obstructed by surplus males lead to heightened social inequality and political volatility.

Some of these analyses have been disputed or even controversial. Kanazawa's "first law of inter-group conflict" theory, in particular, has been challenged by scholars unable to replicate his findings. In general, research that links polygyny closely to various negative social and political outcomes is vulnerable to one particular critique: this linkage is ambiguous, and the direction of causation hard to infer, for the simple reason that women are not randomly selected into polygynous marriages. Rather, polygynous marriages tend to attract women who command less bargaining power and agency before even entering the marriage market. Put differently, polygyny depends on the existence of already-subjugated women even as it contributes to women's subjugation. Historically speaking, with the exception of imperial families giving their daughters in marriage to kings and emperors, it is likely that most women entering into plural marriages have come from less fortunate backgrounds (see Chapter 4). Rather than being viewed as the root cause of violence, therefore, polygyny might be better understood as a proxy for patriarchy, misogyny, and gender inequality.

A related criticism pertains to the assumption that unmarried men in high-polygyny societies are motivated to participate in risky, violent behaviors because they understand themselves to be shut out of marriage markets with no prospects to find wives or father children. Ethnographic research in a number of high-polygyny contexts has found a pervasive perception that females naturally outnumber males in the population—a perception that has been dubbed "the myth of female overpopulation." Bachelors in these settings tend to perceive their marriage prospects as delayed rather than denied, and frequently understand this delay as a natural fact rather than something imposed upon them by their elders.

A more significant critique of the polygyny and warfare literature concerns what is perhaps the core assumption made in this research—namely, that unbalanced sex ratios lead to sexual competition and violence. As we saw in the case of Senegal in Chapter 3, the mere existence of high levels of polygyny by no means excludes significant numbers of men from the marriage market. Moreover, scholars have identified some cases where sex ratios skewed toward men have not increased sexual competition, and others where sex ratios skewed toward women led to harmful outcomes. In light of such findings, the "more males, more violence" prediction that continually arises with respect to polygyny should be handled with considerable caution.

SHOULD POLYGYNY BE BANNED?

For many scholars, evidence of polygyny's harm to women in particular and to society in general has led to the conclusion that it should be abolished. Removing polygyny as a legal marital option, they have decided, would have the most direct effect in mitigating or undoing various forms of social oppression. "Policymakers would have to change multiple laws across multiple domains," write Rose McDermott and Jonathan Cowden, "to exert as much of an effect on these negative outcomes toward women and children as could be accomplished by the abolition of polygyny." Michèle Tertilt has similarly argued that polygyny should be outlawed specifically as a way to fight poverty.

In the second half of the twentieth century, a number of international legal conventions emerged with the aim of promoting human rights, including women's rights. Many of these conventions frame polygyny as a problem. The United Nations Convention on the Elimination of All Forms of Discrimination Against Women (CEDAW), for example, adopted by the UN General Assembly in

1979 and subsequently ratified by 189 countries, calls for abolishing all discriminatory marriage laws, and a CEDAW implementation committee ruled in 1994 that "polygamous marriage contravenes a woman's right to equality with men, and can have such serious emotional and financial consequences for her and her dependents that such marriages ought to be discouraged and prohibited." Similarly, the Protocol of the African Charter on Human and People's Rights on the Rights of Women in Africa, also known as the Maputo Protocol, adopted by the African Union in 2003, sets out monogamy as "the preferred form of marriage."

There is little indication, however, that such legal encouragement of monogamy has spurred widespread moves to ban polygyny, even by governments that have ratified these conventions. Some 49 African states have signed the Maputo Protocol, for example, yet polygynous marriage remained legal in at least 33 of them as of 2020.

In countries where polygyny has long been socially accepted, official bans have a mixed record of success. As we have seen, both Türkiye and Tunisia legally abolished plural marriage in the middle decades of the twentieth century. Polygyny has remained a rare and largely underground practice in both of these countries. By contrast, the West African states of Côte d'Ivoire and Guinea passed laws abolishing polygyny in the 1960s, yet plural marriage has persisted informally in both countries, which rarely enforced its criminalization. To make its laws more consistent with social practice, Guinea dropped its ban in 2016 and adopted a new law recognizing and regulating polygynous marriage three years later.

Efforts to restrict polygyny without banning it also have an uneven track record. In a number of countries including Bangladesh, Iraq, Malaysia, Morocco, and Syria, husbands must prove to a judge that they have the means to maintain additional wives before they are permitted to marry again, and polygynous husbands can be criminally charged for failing to treat their wives equitably. In the sub-Saharan African countries where the largest numbers of polygynous marriages can be found, however, few legal restrictions on the practice exist, and even fewer are reliably enforced.

CONCLUSION: WHAT TO DO ABOUT POLYGYNY AND INEQUALITY?

While there is no scholarly consensus on whether polygyny *causes* inequality and conflict, researchers agree that a strong *correlation* exists between polygyny and inequality, particularly gender inequality. Debates continue as to the nature of this correlation and what it suggests for public policy. If polygyny is, as Rose McDermott and colleagues would have it, "one of the most parsimonious reasons for poor state outcomes, low rates of economic development, and horrific human security," then there are good reasons to demand its abolition. But it is unclear how to implement a successful legal ban in societies where polygyny remains concordant with longstanding social norms. Legal reform alone is likely to have limited results in lowering inequality and discrimination against women, particularly in countries with weak state institutions and low state capacity—a problem afflicting most of the countries with high polygyny rates. If scholars like Valerie Hudson are right that polygyny is merely one component of a structural dynamic of patriarchy and misogyny, then it would be wise to address inequality through broad efforts to educate girls and eliminate legal discrimination rather than targeted bans of polygyny.

FURTHER READING

Economist Michèle Tertilt's article "Polygyny, Women's Rights, and Development," published in the *Journal of the European Economic Association* (2006), makes the case that abolishing polygyny, as well as arranged marriage, would constitute an effective tool for reducing poverty. Her analysis of economic data suggests that "enforcing monogamy" would have the most significant effects, though she makes no proposal for how monogamy could be enforced.

Political scientist Rose McDermott, in *The Evils of Polygyny: Evidence of Its Harm to Women, Men, and Society* (2018) uses a large dataset drawn from 176 countries to argue that polygyny drives a range of negative social outcomes from poverty to armed conflict. McDermott and colleagues find a pattern of instability and violence in poor countries which they associate with polygynous marriage.

Political scientists Valerie Hudson, Donna Lee Bowen, and Perpetua Lynne Nielsen, in their book *The First Political Order: How Sex Shapes Governance and National Security Worldwide* (2020), adopt a wider perspective on plural marriage and women's disempowerment. In countries where polygyny rates are high, the authors identify a "Patrilineal/Fraternal Syndrome," a concept they use to describe an interlocking web of institutions, processes, and norms designed to subordinate women and consolidate power among male kin. Unlike McDermott, these authors situate polygyny not as the primary culprit for negative social outcomes but as an important component of the Patrilineal/Fraternal Syndrome. Their argument draws from the same dataset as McDermott and from a broad scholarly literature on gender inequality.

BIBLIOGRAPHY

Hudson, V., Bowen, D. L., and Nielsen, P. L. (2020). *The first political order: How sex shapes governance and national security worldwide*. Columbia University Press.

McDermott, R. (2018). *The evils of polygyny: Evidence of its harm to women, men, and society*. Oxford University Press.

Tertilt, M. (2006). Polygyny, women's rights, and development. *Journal of the European Economic Association*, 4(2–3),523–530.

6

POLYANDRY

A CULTURAL ODDITY?

Historically speaking, polyandry—or one woman married to many husbands—has been an unusual family arrangement. It was viewed as a family unit best adapted for survival in high-altitude regions with scarce natural resources and unpredictable life-threatening conditions. In Bhutan, until 1914, it was the preferred, albeit not the only, marriage system. In Sri Lanka, until it was banned by the British in 1859, polyandry was common. Julius Caesar found it was common among the ancient Britons. In ancient Rome, there are reports of mature married women begging the Senate to legitimize marriage between a woman and two men. In India, several small ethnic groups practicing polyandry justify the practice as mirroring the behavior of Draupadi, a female character in the classic *Mahabharata*, who married five brothers and diligently worked to maintain a harmonious family. In contemporary India, polyandry is tolerated but not encouraged or celebrated and it remains widespread among the Himalayan Sherpas. In the western Judeo-Christian heritage, there are no examples of women married to more than one man, and the practice is unknown in the Jewish tradition. Today, most Christian denominations strongly advocate monogamous marriage, with a passage from Paul's epistles explicitly forbidding polyandry: "For a married woman is bound by law to her husband while he lives … So then, if she marries another man while her husband is alive, she will be called an adulteress" (Romans 7: 2–3).

DOI: 10.4324/9781003628729-7

Clearly, polygyny (or one man and numerous wives) was easier, due to its historic frequency, to comprehend, if not always approve, as a marital arrangement. In contrast, polyandry has been viewed as a cultural oddity. The puzzlement among Americans, Muslims, and others regarding polyandrous marriage may arise from underlying gender assumptions that women are monogamous-oriented and do not, unless coerced, become sexually involved with numerous men. The strength of this conviction rests on the belief that women prefer monogamy and anything that undermines this "natural" state is a troubling outlier.

Anthropological research has found, however, that the issue of what is and is not the "ideal" marital form is more complicated. In most communities that tolerate polyandry there is wide variation, with some organized around a polyandrous ethos, others preferring polygynous (one man several wives) arrangements, while others prefer monogamy. The point to remember is that family formation is fluid and varied and seldom absolute. We now know that marriage around the globe often assumes many forms in response to extenuating factors.

HOW RARE IS POLYANDRY?

A comprehensive survey of 1231 societies listed in the 1980 Ethnographic Atlas categorized 186 societies as monogamous, 1041 as polygynous (occasional or frequent), and 4 as practicing classical polyandry. However, revisionist research (discussed below) has found support for "nonclassical" polyandry, which is less rare than formerly thought. The best-known region where polyandry is an established practice is the Plateau of Tibet which shares geographical border with India, Nepal, the Tibet Autonomous Region of China. A 1988 survey of 753 Tibetan families found that approximately 13 percent practiced polyandry. Beyond Tibet, only a handful of other communities have been documented as maintaining similar marital arrangements. These include several ethnic minority groups in southern China (e.g., the Moso), inhabitants of the Marquesas Islands in the South Pacific, and a few scattered localities in sub-Saharan Africa, such as Nigeria's Erigwith and communities surrounding the Lake Region of Central Africa, where women may be married to multiple husbands. Taken together, it is estimated that only around 4 percent of global cultures practice some form of classical polyandry.

WHY CLASSICAL OR FORMAL POLYANDRY?

Classical—or formal—polyandry refers to socially recognized and institutionalized marriages in which one woman is married to two or more men, most commonly brothers. Unlike informal or episodic arrangements, classical polyandry is embedded in local kinship systems, inheritance rules, and moral expectations, and it functions as a durable household strategy rather than an experimental or ideologically driven form of intimacy.

Polyandry usually assumes one of four forms: (1) fraternal polyandry (in which a woman is married to a group of brothers) and (2) non-fraternal polyandry (in which unrelated men agree to marry one woman), (3) informal (or ad hoc) polyandry, and (4) mixed polyandry/polygyny. The institutional or classical polyandrous marriage is often, but not always, between one woman and two or more men who are usually brothers. It is a formalized arrangement with a recognized sexual division of labor that carries with it acceptable expectations and individual rights. It is assumed that men occupy higher social status over women, with everyone having mutual obligations to each other through a commitment to work for the betterment of the larger family. It is a serious contract where usually a group of brothers agrees to contribute their labor, sexual interest, and child support. Each member of the fraternal group, regardless of age, is ideally regarded as equivalent and more esteemed than daughters. The governing folk ideology holds that no brother can claim exclusive rights to the wife. Nor can anyone claim exclusive rights to the land, houses, or cattle. The incoming wife must consider all her husbands to be equivalent and instruct the children to address all her husbands as "father." She is also expected to perform domestic chores for all the brothers, to treat them fairly, in sexual and other matters, be open and willingly to procreate. Similarly, polygynous men instruct their children to address all their wives as "mother."

Although polyandry is anchored in an egalitarian ethos, there are still inequities. The eldest brother holds certain authority in the family and more opportunity to father children in the early years of the marriage. Brothers who are no longer willing to collectively share their labor and incomes must terminate the marriage. The marriage contract can be broken by either party, but the children remain with the father and not the mother. Fraternal polyandrous marriage, between biologically related brothers, tends to be the most stable. When unrelated men form a non-fraternal family, being unrelated, they are in more explicit competition for status and reproductive benefit. The dissatisfaction is evident in repeated findings that it is men more than women that defect from their polyandrous marriage to marry monogamously. The man usually finds a new wife, or just as often a mistress and they live together as an unmarried couple.

The effort to form a pair bond is not without difficulty. It often leads to the division of collectively owned family land, a process that frequently results in the family's impoverishment. In response, some members establish client relationships with wealthier families, while others migrate to nearby townships, where they seek employment as common laborers.

Informal polyandry, unlike fraternal polyandry (where a woman will receive several husbands simultaneously), expands in sequence when the wife accepts, often staggering, one husband after another. The ad hoc form is amazingly flexible. It may or may not be organized around a ranked hierarchical system where one husband is considered primary and is allotted certain rights and privileges not awarded to a secondary or non-primary husband, such as fathering a child. Informal polyandry usually begins as a dyadic affair that expands to include other husbands. It may take the form of "visiting husbands" in groups like the Nayar in South India and Mosuo communities in Southwest China. With visiting husbands, women have brief or long-term partners who visit them in their parents' homes.

The Nayar of southern India are an intriguing oddity. Around puberty, a Nayar girl is ritually granted the status of a married "adult" woman, though she does not enter into a formal, co-residential marriage. Once recognized as an adult, she is socially permitted to engage in a succession of visiting lovers. Outside observers often characterized this arrangement as polyandrous; however, it more closely resembles what would today be described as polyamory (see Chapter 7). Importantly, this system did not eliminate concerns about paternity. Rather, questions of fatherhood were accommodated within the matrilineal descent framework, which located primary social identity and inheritance in the woman's lineage, which served as the center of her life, whose members live together and cooperate in child rearing.

THE ORIGINS OF CLASSICAL OR FORMAL POLYANDRY

Anthropological evidence indicates that classical polyandry arose under a distinctive constellation of ecological, economic, and demographic pressures. It is most consistently documented in high-altitude or resource-scarce regions—most notably across the Himalayan belt (Tibet, Ladakh, Nepal, Bhutan)—where arable land is limited, climatic conditions are harsh, and household survival depends on maintaining consolidated estates. In such contexts, fraternal polyandry serves as a mechanism to prevent the fragmentation of landholdings that would otherwise result from successive generations of monogamous marriages and partible inheritance.

Societies practicing classical polyandry are overwhelmingly agricultural. It is a marriage system that arises out of a response to an imbalanced sex ratio, adult male mortality, male absenteeism, economic fragility and, for established polyandrous communities. Much ink has been spilled in trying to identify the reasons behind why people prefer polyandry vs polygyny or monogamy. Why is the classical polyandrous family located in a few regions and absent in others? Different explanations have been advanced to account for its appearance in one locality but have been less successful in accounting for its appearance or disappearance in another region.

At its core, polyandry represents a solution to a structural problem: how to reconcile population continuity with economic viability in environments where resources cannot be easily expanded. By keeping brothers within a single marital unit, families preserve land, livestock, and labor within one corporate household. All husbands contribute economically, while the wife manages domestic production and reproduction, thereby stabilizing the household across generations. This arrangement reduces competition among male siblings and minimizes the risk of downward mobility that might accompany household fission.

The more prevalent explanation is environmental. It is the scarcity of environmental resources such as arable land which compels a family to engage in a more restrictive inheritance rather than equally dividing its limited land between all the offspring. Fraternal polyandry is a response to retain intergenerational wealth that grows out of a need to survive life in an environment with scarce resources (e.g., arable land). This factor, more than any others, compels a family to embrace a restrictive inheritance custom rather than practice an equitable distribution of family resources amongst all the male offspring. Keeping the brothers together and united through marriage with a sole wife produces only one set of heirs per generation. It is a subset that ideally remains together and, thus, protects and retains the family's valuable land.

The incorporation of the brothers into a marital unit reduces reproductive conflict and keeps the family property intact. The family's motivation is like that of the nineteenth-century European primogeniture custom, whereby the eldest son inherits the family estate while younger brothers are urged to seek their fortune in military service or in the clergy. Another motivation for the formation of polyandrous families arises out of an anxiety over individuals wanting to maintain their social position linked with the relative size of their family's land estate. Here is one reason behind the Nyinbans (of Tibet) stressing that they need men's labor more than their procreation ability. Because aristocratic titles were linked to the size of a family's agricultural estate, there were negative consequences to terminating a family's land holdings. Amongst the Tibetan priestly class, it was the threat of loss of social status that made individuals reluctant to divide their family's property and therefore made them reluctant to live monogamously.

Polyandrous communities in the Tibetan Plateau tend to be stratified: wealthier families have more arable land and prefer polyandry, while poorer families with less land practice monogamy. Paradoxically, the larger the fraternal sibling group, the more the polyandrous marriage creeps toward personal dissatisfaction and disorder. Why? It has to do with the limitations of the human lifespan. Because brothers are different ages, fraternal polyandry can create an awkward situation for a younger brother.

Imagine a boy who is five years old when his older brother marries, so that by the time he is in his late twenties his wife may be in her later thirties or older, creating a reproductive disjunction between relative youth and middle age. This emotional ambiguity and biological constraint contribute to the younger brother's push to divide the family's property.

A polyandrous husband may also experience emotional angst over whether his wife cares or loves all her husbands equally. The issue of emotional equity is not unique to the polyandrous family: Fundamentalist Mormons' wives repeatedly ask their husband whether he loves all his wives the same. The husband, if politically astute, replies "yes." But it is a qualified yes: as men will admit to close friends, they don't really feel the same way for each of their wives. A similar psychological process exists in a polyandrous family. In the end it is difficult to love everyone equally. There is always a "favorite" husband or wife (see Chapter 4).

Other researchers note that another factor explaining the draw of polyandry could be the frequent absence, for long periods, of men from the household which would allow extramarital mating opportunities. It is also not unknown for a wife to enter an illicit sexual affair, which can threaten family unity. One way to neutralize a woman's potential sexual exploratory activities is to marry her to a set of brothers who can monopolize her time and attention—polyandry, in this context, can function as a patriarchal surveillance strategy. This is not always an effective strategy. However, it does reveal the presence of an acute anxiety over parental certainty.

Another form of polyandry is a combination of polyandry and polygyny, often referred to as double-polyandrous/polygynous union, in which a woman marries several men simultaneously while the same men are married to other women. This is a variation of informal polyandry. It can be based on an egalitarian understanding where all husbands are equal in status and receive the same rights and privileges, or it can be a subset of the prevailing ranked hierarchy that limits some men's privileges. In a few northern Nigerian regions and in some northern Cameroonian villages, it is not usual for a polyandrous woman's husband to also marry another woman living in a different village. Why is this? The double-polyandrous union is more a marital alliance than an emotional bond. It links the interests of rival groups not individuals in a "contractual" arrangement that furthers the groups over an individual's interest.

A related, albeit different, form of marital union, sometimes referred to as a secondary marriage, arises when a married man or woman cohabits with someone other than their spouse, but later accepts a new, albeit secondary, spouse who may or may not replace her first husband as the primary source of emotional satisfaction. A polyandrous marriage is grounded in a publicized commitment to forming a marital unit. This distinguished it from an extramarital affair, which is usually conducted in secret and devoid of obligations or normative expectations. It is the public commitment to the marriage, involving restrictive sexual access to specific people along with other family-centered expectations and "rights," that distinguishes institutionalized polyandry from informal polyandry, or a sexual affair. The ambiguity over whether an ongoing affair that is not institutionalized constitutes the presence of a "secondary" husband is the essence of the debate over whether the arrangement is polyandrous or something else.

SHARED PATERNITY—INFORMAL POLYANDRY?

There are societies that believe a successful pregnancy requires multiple acts of sexual intercourse from different men. It assumes a healthy child requires more than one father-creator who is sexually involved with the mother, perceives the offspring as quasi-kin and will assist the child in the future or whenever needed. Anthropologist Stephen Beckerman identified 20 Amazonian tribal societies that insisted a child needs more than one father. He labelled this orientation shared paternity, which Katherine Starkweather and Raymon Hames would later argue is a nonclassical form of informal polyandry. Beckerman conducted research amongst the Amazonian Bari who believe a healthy child requires a partial or supplemental father who through repeated sexual intercourse with one woman helped in the child's formation. His investigation found a Bari child 16 percent more likely than a single-fathered child to survive to the age of 15, probably due to improved nutrition an extra "father" can bring to the family. Having multiple "fathers" protects children among the Ache foragers of eastern Paraguay from domestic violence, the main cause of infant and child mortality. Clearly, frequent sexual intercourse with the same woman draws men closer to the woman and more open to rendering support to an offspring associated with that interaction. Does this relationship constitute another variation on nonclassical polyandry? After childbirth, there is no expectation of a woman's continued sexual availability, it appears the relationship ends with the birth of a child, and there is no property to protect or inherit. However, there is a long-term relationship established between the child and the secondary "father." This suggests that the Bari have conceptualized the supportive relationship as something beyond a sexual tryst. It does involve an intergenerational transfer based on practical guidance and occasional material support. In many respects, the institutionalization of "secondary" fathers is comparable to the Latin American system of godparenthood, in that both establish enduring bonds between distinct households. The key difference, however, is that in the Amazonian cases these inter-household ties also entail explicit obligations to the woman's child.

BUT IS IT AN ANTHROPOLOGICAL FANTASY?

It has been suggested that the pair bond cannot be a human universal if the biological father can be shared or easily substituted. Some have insisted that the Bari and related Amazonian "tribal" groups represent an earlier era where humans rejected the pair bond in favor of unattached "group sex." This is a position that anthropologist Warren Shapiro insists is wrong. He points out that it is found in only one Amazonian population, which does not satisfy the geographical requirement for the behavior having a greater antiquity.

Offering a counter qualification, Kathrine Starkweather and Raymond Hames' (2012) investigation identified 53 small-scale or nonclassical societies around the globe (including North America and South America) that practiced a form of partial paternity. In all societies, husbands were ranked differently—the first husband was ranked as primary with the second husband serving as a supplemental, supportive resource. The authors found that shared paternity—a variation of informal polyandry—is more widely practiced, albeit organized around a hierarchical delegated responsibility that varied depending upon whether the husband was deemed primary or secondary. Their research suggests that when it comes to survival, women are immensely pragmatic and more than willing to exchange sex for assistance and resources.

What is equally of significance is the reluctance of Bari women to engage in sexual exchanges with strangers. These women prefer an established sexual bond with one or two men, but rarely with four or more men. This suggests that sexual involvement remains for women an emotionally charged activity that most women are comfortable conceptualizing and sustaining as a quasi-pair bond relationship with men who are in good agreement to cooperate and tolerate each other's presence.

A historical example of a shared paternity relationship comes from Qing China. In eighteenth- and nineteenth-century (late Qing) China, there was a practice whereby a wife took into her home another man or sexual partner for a fixed period who would provide additional income. This arrangement was referred to as "Getting a husband to support a husband." Under Qing law, it was illegal to have more than one "husband." Most villagers did not practice this, but some "adopted" for a while another "husband" to bring in additional income that insured survival. The historian Mathew Sommer's study of Qing legal code found numerous instances in which the wife pushed her legally married husband to either sell her to a more successful married or unmarried man who could provide sufficient food for her and her children or invite another unmarried man into their family. For example, in one case, a husband told his wife:

> If we lose this man, and don't bring him into our family, then who are we going to find who can help us? I've already acknowledged him as family ... if you don't obey me, then I'll die here, I refuse to go on.

Reluctantly, she agreed. Another legal case recorded an impoverished wife's anguish as she took the lead in bringing into her family another "husband." She harassed her husband verbally, complaining bitterly to her family about her husband's poverty and incompetence. She added: "I saw he could not support a wife and that if I stayed with him, I would end up starving to death."

Do these Qing dynasty examples constitute polyandrous marriage? If everyone agreed to this arrangement, a period was set in which the arrangement would last before the contract was terminated. Sometimes this resulted in the woman leaving with the new husband, other times she decided to remain with her first husband.

Whether she left or stayed depended upon "feelings" she had or did not have for men involved in her newly formed, albeit secret, marriage. The negotiated "relationships" were conducted within a monogamous framework that did not formally recognize secondary "husbands." In the end, this form of unconventional "marriage" arose out of extreme poverty and not prurient sexual interest or a romantic longing. Chinese women, like people everywhere, are active agents who use sexuality to develop or sustain long-term bonds that enhance their survival. It often arises out of an ad hoc situational strategy that may or may not result in a formalized exchange. Whatever form it takes, it is organized around acquiring additional resources for a woman and her offspring. How do we interpret this behavior?

Anthropology has always had a bias of assigning one overarching ideology to a community that ignores the presence of alternative practices. Starkweather and Hames found evidence that some, but not all women, in a variety of non-Amazonian societies are open to forging alternative "marital" bonds. Their finding does not mean there was an earlier primal era where men and women preferred group marriage over a pair bond arrangement. It does suggest, however, that the development of shared paternity or a polyandrous relationship may be a temporal survival adaptation that is entered into under duress and not out of a desire for adventure, sexual excitement, or spiritual fulfillment. In coding human variation, it remains essential to remember that in every society there are ethnographic intermediates between single paternity, semi-partial paternity, shared paternity, and classical polyandry.

WHO'S YOUR DADDY?

Nyinba (of Tibet) husbands try to track and allocate paternity. Given the plurality of sexual encounters, it is difficult, but not impossible, to know who a child's actual father is—but everyone wants to know all the same. Nimba are forever speculating who their father is. Given this, men often suspect women will try to target one husband or brother whom she wants to take with her if the family's land is later partitioned or perhaps to intend to lobby for a partition and keep their child with them. To this end, polyandrous families are forever speculating over who is a child's genitor. This can arise out of harmless fun and be based on casual curiosity. In fraternal polyandry, the children are often, but not always, said to be descended from the eldest brother alone, while in other families, fatherhood is established through invoking a normative statement that the children are thought to have descended from all the husbands equally. In other cases, it is understood but reluctantly commented upon when a wife tries to organize her fertility cycle in such a way that her "favorite" husband to whom she is most attracted has the inside track to her reproduction. Other times, especially if the wife begins to publicly speculate about who a child resembles, her raising the subject of a child's paternity could be viewed as a sign that she wants to leave the larger family for a more preferred husband with whom she has formed an emotional bond.

Evolutionary psychologists suggest there is a downside to shared paternity. Sexual jealousy is more frequent than initially reported. Sexual jealousy is a human universal that most people find difficult to eliminate. Co-husbands express jealousy and competition in various ways, including earning capacity, working capacity, physique, clothing, food, and public status. The husbands try to keep physical distance whenever possible and thus avoid triggering sexual jealousy. What is remarkable is that some individuals can mute their reactions and try to "work" within the prevailing folk ideology that encourages detachment and toleration for the sexual complexities of living in a pluralistic marriage.

However, sexual rivalry between fraternal brothers is more the exception. Fraternal brothers' families resemble a sororal family (i.e., natal sisters), where sexual jealousy is more easily muted. This does not mean there is no sexual competition. It does mean that there will be, at times, an absence of mutual compatibility which can lead to the wife ignoring, rejecting, and withdrawing from her older first husband in favor of a younger (but not prepuberty husband) whom she regards as more physically attractive and who may share similar generational understandings. Still, there can be a discrepancy between the folk ideal of sexual tolerance and the experience of sexual jealousy. Nancy Levine, in her classic account *The Dynamics of Polyandry: Kinship, Domesticity and Population in the Tibetan Border*, reports that sexual jealousy is managed through having a regular sleeping schedule, like many polygynous families, of which everyone is aware and which enables the other husbands to be physically unavailable. The management is made easier when a wife's co-husbands do not or are unable to visit. Because "husbands" may be pastoralists, work as temporary day laborers, or as low-ranking government officials stationed outside their home village, avoidance of potential sexual awkwardness is easier to manage.

Sexual jealousy remains an unvoiced but persistent concern among brothers, who nonetheless remain diligent in establishing a workable "visiting" system that affords each husband a degree of sexual privacy. The management of sexual access, however, does not always proceed smoothly. It is not uncommon for some brothers to become dissatisfied with the sharing arrangement and to seek alternative sexual or emotional bonds with other women.

Levine tells a story about three Nyinba brothers who decided to bring other women into the family only to realize their land was insufficient and too marginal to support everyone. This resulted in the brothers terminating their plural marriage. In another case, three brothers sharing a wife agreed that they were too many to share a single woman. The realization they could no longer satisfactorily manage their sexual behavior and reproductive interests resulted in the termination of the plural family in favor of monogamy. The desire to form a dyadic bond compels them to go against their long-term material interest in keeping their family's land together in favor of their individual reproductive interest and emotional needs. It is a sentiment to form a dyadic bond that fundamentalist Mormon polygynous men often experience but are reluctant to acknowledge.

Fundamentalist men's reluctance stems from their deep-seated commitment to a cosmology that regards plural—or, in their terms, "noble love"—as superior to what they view as the more conventional dyadic or romantic love bond. The value placed on noble love, defined as equal love among all family members, is promoted as a livable ideal through church services, religious schooling, family outings, and extended conversations with a visiting anthropologist. Given the community's dedication to noble love, it is striking how common "favoritism," or affectionate preference for one wife over others, proves to be in everyday practice. In many ways, the unvoiced acknowledgment of a favored wife functions as a public secret—one that paradoxically contributes to the community's capacity to sustain itself as a viable alternative to mainstream society.

Greetanjali Tiwari's research among the Kimmaur, who live in the Himalayas of India, found that local wives readily acknowledged: "The life of a wife is emotionally challenging. As a polyandrous wife she must be careful in voicing her disapproval of a husband's actions—to do otherwise can be construed as favoritism." Thus, she added: "a more aloof persona is required." The persona may help but it does not necessarily result in everyone's satisfaction. For example, a 20-something Kimmaur man acknowledged an uneasiness about how he became involved in a polyandrous marriage. He recalled:

> I did not choose any of the wives ... although my brothers did obtain my consent before marrying. I was too young to be a husband to my elder brother's first wife and when I became age-appropriate to marry, my youthful new wife told me she did not like me ... I find polyandry too difficult for me—I think the polyandrous family's overall success depends on the wife.

In effect, the wife in the role of emotional manager can strengthen or undermine the plural marriage.

The polyandrous wife occupies the center of the family and should be regarded as the family's emotional manager. It is a crucial and most difficult familial role. She is aware of her responsibility to effectively manage her husband's emotional angst over whether he is loved and equally valued. A woman's family broke up when she declined to tell a husband she loved him as much as his brothers. She explained:

> I tried to love both the husbands equally, but it got harder. My older husband fathered five of my children, but the two men [i.e., her co-husbands] are so different. My older husband lived far away and grew to prefer his independence. My younger husband is so gentle he listens to me and does what I say. I can trust him ... I am a lucky woman.

However, she admitted that, seeing how her other husbands had promised but quickly ceased to provide economic assistance and support, she prefers to live monogamously.

The fragility of polyandrous marriages often arises from material scarcity and from emotional dissatisfaction generated by the sharing of a common spouse. This does not mean, however, that few families are able to find satisfaction within polyandrous arrangements. On the contrary, researchers have consistently reported that many families are able to create and sustain workable forms of marital satisfaction. The more difficult question concerns what is meant by "satisfaction." For some participants, contentment is derived primarily from the fulfillment of role obligations, with or without strong emotional attachment. Others, however, desire deeper affective bonds and experience intense dissatisfaction with the necessity of sharing a spouse. As in all family systems, there is considerable variation among individuals. Identifying the tension points within a given family system thus helps reveal the presence of competing voices and often unspoken values that shape marital experience.

CONCLUSION

From a comparative and evolutionary–anthropological perspective, women's participation in polyandry is best understood not as a single "benefit" but as a bundle of contingent advantages, most of which are structural and pragmatic rather than romantic. Across ethnographic cases, women tend to *gain security and stability* more than emotional fulfillment.

Because polyandrous households are wealthier and have higher socioeconomic status relative to monogamous families, it may be beneficial to enter a polyandrous marriage where there is material support and personal protection. The risk of death is ever present, and it is often wise to retain others who can and are willing to offer support to household members. Polyandrous marriages mute the chances of a dire widowhood and help ensure women's survival. Given this potential benefit, there is a tradeoff where a woman sacrifices her reproductive interest, contributes valuable labor in exchange for material, and, at times, emotional support.

Women also benefit from stable provisioning rather than dependence on a single male earner. The family stability often enhances the wife's authority over household management, as she becomes the linchpin around which the emotional and reproductive lives of family members are organized.

In societies where polyandry is normative, a polyandrous wife gains prestige as a household manager who mediates relationships among brothers (or her husbands) and helps sustain family cohesion. Children, in turn, may benefit from the involvement of multiple adult males or paternal figures, while paternity ambiguity can reduce favoritism and encourage collective investment.

Yet these advantages coexist with significant emotional constraints. Polyandry may be socially functional, but it is often emotionally costly. Sustaining an exclusive, emotionally intense dyadic relationship is difficult within a polyandrous system. Over time, emotional hierarchies frequently emerge, and when such hierarchies become pronounced, they can undermine cooperation and precipitate the collapse of the polyandrous family.

Social class also plays a role in shaping a woman's life satisfaction. Research has repeatedly found that at the symbolic level, low-status women in polyandrous marriages are regarded as second-class citizens lacking authority over men. However, at the everyday family level, they have enormous power to influence their husbands' willingness to remain in a polyandrous marriage. Given that men are drawn to and need affectionate reassurance, the sole wife in a plural marriage—much like the queen on a chessboard—has enormous power, even as she remains confined in a society that symbolically regards women as inferior to men.

A polyandrous marriage may benefit a woman through providing access to greater wealth. Because polyandrous households are wealthier and have higher socioeconomic status relative to monogamous families, it may be beneficial to enter a polyandrous marriage where there is material support and personal protection. The risk of death is everpresent, and it is often wise to retain others who are willing to offer support. Polyandrous marriages lessen the chances of a dire widowhood and help ensure a woman's well-being. Given this potential benefit there is a tangible tradeoff where a woman sacrifices her reproductive interest, contributes valuable labor in exchange for material, and, at times, emotional support. It is seldom an easy exchange, but neither is living in a high-altitude environment with limited resources while managing a plural family with discordant voices.

FURTHER READING

Polyandry's global rarity makes it a somewhat obscure topic with little research (particularly book-length studies) devoted to it. One notable exception is Nancy Levine's book *The Dynamics of Polyandry: Kinship, Domesticity and Population on the Tibetan Border* (1988), the most complete ethnographic account of lived experience within a polyandrous family. One important scholarly article is Melvyn Goldstein's "Stratification, Polyandry, and Family Structure in Central Tibet" (1971), a concise account of the material factors influencing individuals' decisions to enter and remain in polyandrous families. Another is Katherine Starkweather and Raymond Hames' "A Survey of Non-Classical Polyandry," published in *Human Nature* (2012); this groundbreaking study revealed the global prevalence of polyandrous relationships to be greater than previously understood.

BIBLIOGRAPHY

Goldstein, M. C. (1971). Stratification, polyandry, and family structure in central Tibet. *Southwestern Journal of Anthropology*, 27(1), 64–74.

Levine, N. (1988). *The dynamics of polyandry: Kinship, domesticity and population on the Tibetan border*. University of Chicago Press.

Starkweather, K., and Hames, R. (2012). A survey of non-classical polyandry. *Human Nature*, 23(2), 149–172.

7

POLYAMORY

EXPERIMENTING WITH "FREE LOVE"

Throughout the 1960s and 1970s, it was common to find in American college dormitories male students exchanging, with earnest commentary, a 1966 novel entitled *The Harrad Experiment*. The book suggested that the ideal romantic–sexual relationship was not found in a pair bond but rather in a plural love arrangement involving multiple partners. *The Harrad Experiment* centered on one man and his several girlfriends, each with distinct personalities and degrees of sexual attractiveness. The author apparently never considered the possibility that a plural arrangement could also involve one woman with multiple male partners. The novel implied that, at least for men, "marital contentment" was best achieved through men's emotional and sexual variety. For 18-year-olds, this was an exciting prospect. Fifty years later, a new generation of college students remains enamored with the possibility of forming polyamorous—or polyamour—relationship, which many view as an intriguing alternative to the conventional pair bond model.

Even two generations ago, students' openness to an alternative to a monogamous marriage was not new. Monogamous marriage has a long history of individuals questioning its validity, often captured in the mantra, "there must be something better than this." Paradoxically, such doubts have been most pronounced in places and periods strongly associated with monogamy and the nuclear family—modern societies of Western Europe and North America. The eighteenth-century French philosopher Denis Diderot pondered whether it was unnatural to love only one person forever. His

DOI: 10.4324/9781003628729-8

reflections anticipated the Western European reading public's—especially educated women's—growing resistance to forced or arranged marriages. In their place, reformers promoted marital choice, while more radical thinkers insisted that the better ideal was "free love without entanglements." For these activists, "free love" represented a new individuality, freedom of choice, and independence from the constraints of an antiquated social order.

Across the ensuing centuries, the appeal of sexual freedom—and its association with personal growth—retained a persistent allure. Nineteenth-century experimental communes, emerging primarily in North America, insisted that the problems of "modern" living stemmed from the limitations and restrictions inherent in the monogamous family. The Oneida, Owenites, and Fourierists, among others, viewed the nuclear family as an institution that should be discarded. In its place, members were encouraged to engage in consensual non-monogamy, which they believed would free individuals from normative constraints that limited emotional and personal development. These communities imagined themselves as pioneers of a utopian future, encapsulated in their millenarian optimism: "with us begins a new world."

Fast forward to the twentieth century, and we once again find the clarion call for redefining marriage through rejecting monogamous marriage with all its inherent limitations. This call has generally appealed most strongly to educated urban dwellers in Western Europe and North America. In the 1950s, one such group was composed of professionals, most living in New York City, who followed the teachings of Harry Stack Sullivan, a psychoanalyst who argued that sexual repression was responsible for people's angst. He proposed that good health required breaking away from repressive parent-child relationships and monogamous intimacy and instead embracing collective childrearing and sexual variety. His followers in the 1950s formed in rural Oregon and Vermont a "free love" commune that others later brought to New York City in the form of an active urban "commune." They referred to themselves as the Sullivanians, and pursued life satisfaction through discouraging what they saw as the unhealthy romantic dependency of dyadic relationships in favor of sex with multiple familiars (and not strangers). They blamed society's monogamous, nuclear family structure, which they saw as a product of capitalism, for serious mental illness and social breakdown. They insisted that untrammeled sexuality was the secret of happiness and a delightful avenue to personal freedom, self-growth, and life contentment. The group, which had around 500 members, broke up by the early 1990s, with most members disappointed and disillusioned with their utopian experiment, preferring instead to spend more time in exclusive pair bond relationships and parenting their own biological offspring.

These experiments in living anticipated and overlapped with the "baby boomers" 1960s communal trend, which once again questioned the value of monogamous marriage and considered in its place non-obligatory "free love." The sexual liberation advocates of the 1960s and early 1970s believed that monogamy, as an institutional force, undermined personal growth, restricted spiritual rebirth, and promoted gender inequality.

THE LATEST ATTEMPT TO FIND CONTENTMENT IN PLURAL LOVE

Following on the heels of the 1960s "Free Love" communes is the present-day experiment in polyamory or "multiple-lovers" relationships. Polyamory—often framed (alongside polygamy) as "ethical non-monogamy"—is less an alternative marriage system than a lifestyle organized around a philosophy of consensual non-monogamy that values emotional and, at times, sexual relationships with multiple partners. It differs from polygyny (one man and several wives) and polyandry (one woman and several husbands) in its rejection of legalized marital structures and its insistence on the superiority of polyfidelity—practitioners generally dislike the term "plural love," believing it undermines an individual's freedom to alter their relational entanglements.

In its modern American guise, polyamory emerged amid the experiments of 1960s-era counterculture. As detailed in Christopher Gleason's history, *American Poly*, new ideas about ethical non-monogamy took shape as Americans (largely urban, white, and middle-class) felt freed from the constraints of monogamy. Taking inspiration from a wide variety of sources, from Robert Heinlein's science fiction to libertarian ideals to pagan religion, they began trying out practices and rules for non-monogamous relationships. Members of the San Francisco-based Kerista commune were especially influential through the new vocabulary they coined. "Polyfidelity" became a Keristan ideal: members of the commune could have many lovers, so long as they were faithful to the group. They posited "compersion" as an emotional opposite to jealousy for ethical non-monogamists—a feeling of contentment that one could experience in seeing one's lovers enjoy one another. The label "polyamory," however, only came to the fore among ethical non-monogamists in the 1990s through use in online message boards. These days, many people trim the latter term to simply "poly."

Elisabeth Sheff, in her influential book *The Polyamorists Next Door*, reports that polyamorists typically embrace values of social justice, gender equality, autonomy, voluntary cooperation, openness to new romantic possibilities, and a rejection of sexual monogamy. In the United States, polyamory practitioners largely come from the highly educated professional classes and reside primarily in urban areas such as the San Francisco Bay Area, Boston, New York, and Chicago. They represent a narrow cross-section of the American population—cosmopolitan, educated, and socially progressive. Polyamory is particularly attractive to bisexual women, who form a large contingent in European and American communities, although men constitute the majority of philosophically inclined practitioners and are overwhelmingly heterosexual. Importantly, polyamorists—despite their demographic similarities, do not constitute a homogeneous community, nor are they interested in forming a political lobby to promote legal reforms that might make polyamorous living easier. Instead, they prefer to be left alone to practice their chosen lifestyle.

Most practitioners prefer not to conceptualize their relationships through the framework of monogamous commitment—even when, in practice, they live largely monogamous lives with a primary partner. For many, the issue is philosophical: safeguarding the freedom to choose multiple romantic partners rather than restricting oneself to what they view as the constraints of an antiquated monogamous norm. Some adopt what might be termed an "entrepreneurial strategy," keeping multiple relational options open as a hedge against making a permanent emotional commitment. This reluctance does not imply that practitioners cannot or will not form deep emotional bonds; many do. Others establish emotionally and financially committed relationships that resemble "open" marriages.

Crucially, unlike polygynous marriages—typically organized around reproduction, patriarchy, and the consolidation of resources—polyamory emphasizes gender equality and downplays the centrality of reproduction. The contrast is striking between polygyny, embedded in long-standing institutional logics, and polyamory, grounded in personal autonomy, emotional choice, and negotiated flexibility.

LIFESTYLE APPEAL

The polyamory lifestyle appeals, at least as a fantasy ideal, especially to college-educated youth. The US Census 2010 data on single adults reported 20 percent of this highly educated cohort self-reported engaging in consensual non-monogamy. A 2017 study found that Google searches for "polyamory" and "open relationships" rose steadily from January 2006 to December 2015.

By the 2020s, polyamory, as an expressed (though not necessarily lived) personal philosophy, was "hot." Outlets from Medium ("Is Monogamy a Thing of the Past?") to *Psychology Today* ("The New Sexual Revolution") were commenting on the surge of ethically non-monogamous relationships in American society. In a 2021 YouGov poll, about 25 percent of more than 23,000 Americans claimed to be interested in polyamory but had not formed an open relationship. And in 2025, a survey of 1000 British adults showed that 31 percent did not consider monogamy a "realistic" ideal in modern relationships. This sentiment was strongest (42 percent) among respondents aged 24 or younger.

The American college students who are most open to and prefer "relationship freedom" find polyamory appealing, at least as an ideal. European college student attitude surveys report a similar trend. It remains to be seen how many will practice this lifestyle in the long term. For those living the lifestyle it is estimated (no one knows for sure) for the United States there are around 100,000 practitioners. A 2022 Kinsey Institute report found 9 percent of respondents acknowledged they had tried a polyfidelity relationship. It was unclear how many of these were one-off encounters—something to try and move on from, and how many initiated the respondent into an alternative lifestyle that brought greater satisfaction.

This increase is suggestive of an openness to new possibilities that, according to polyamorists, will lead to deeper, richer emotional relationships. Polyamorists' rejection of monogamous life stems from the desire to live an unrestrictive life over which they feel a sense of control, and, thus, not to be limited by sterile monogamous conventions. Much like the 1990s homosexual rights movement, polyamory seeks respectability and its advocates insist they are not equivalent to "swinging" or consensual spousal exchange, nor to a 1970s-style "open marriage" organized around the pursuit of sexual variety for its own sake. Polyamory practitioners challenge this depiction and insist that theirs is a new philosophy that promotes the establishment of richer emotional connections that contribute to personal growth.

The ground rules of polyamory mirror many self-help books that promote the ideal relationship as "pure," which means it is based on trust, intimacy, co-equal decision making, and mutual consent. Individuals have unrestricted freedom to express themselves as sexual beings. To its advocates, the polyamory lifestyle is superior to monogamy in its ability to provide for enhanced empowerment and self-development that blossoms best within a plural relationship network. Some suggest that polyamory relationships work best if they begin as intimate friendships that may or may not become sexual. In time, if participants are willing, this can result in the sexualization of friendship whereby affection and asexual love transform into an erotic romantic relationship. Intimate friendship is an easier way to begin a polyamory relationship and it is consistent with women's evolved imperative to seek signs of partners' stronger emotional investment.

Our fascination with the polyamory lifestyle arises from its challenge to the long-held assumption that we can only find marital satisfaction with one person. Polyamory represents a philosophical challenge to monogamy and the pair bond. Some polyamory advocates insist that heterosexuality is a learned and not a "natural" orientation. They further contend that monogamy is not "normal" but a byproduct of Christianity and capitalism that created a family hierarchy favoring men's interests over women's interests. These advocates believe that humans were never meant to live monogamously and that their own lifestyle stands as a refutation to the claim that humans are a pair bond species. Rather, they contend, we have only been socialized into believing this is so.

Polyamorists appeal to earlier anthropological research that they erroneously claim proves that early humans preferred group marriage over monogamy. This interpretation would suggest that group marriage and not monogamy is the more "natural" institution. Given this finding, the lifestyle could be viewed no longer as a cultural oddity but rather as a return to the more "natural" way of life we have somehow forgotten. It is a claim that has not received much empirical support (discussed below).

The polyamory literature and preliminary empirical research are written as an advocacy essay emphasizing the life-satisfaction gained through creating a polyfidelity union. Many such essays read as the equivalent to a secularized "Sermon on the Mount" promising a greater good that can only come through surrendering the self to wider interpersonal intimacy. For more neutral researchers, this presents a problem: how many people experience what has been promised? We just do not know. Sheff's groundbreaking study provided an overview on the various types of polyfidelity (or enclosed poly unions) sprinkled with delightful quotes that highlighted benefits and problems, especially those involving sexual jealousy. Her primary focus was, however, on the offspring who lived with parent(s) in a polyunit or on similar committed individuals (discussed in Chapter 3).

Recently polyamory, as a viable philosophy of love, has received support from some anthropologists who insist that the pair bond is and has always been a culturally constructed ideal. As we saw in previous chapters, the anthropological record has documented numerous polygynous and polyandrous cultures whose members tolerate or even idealize non-monogamous marriage. From this perspective, efforts at forming complex family/plural love relationships are not an oddity but can be potentially successful. Other scholars disagree, arguing that an impulse to form a pair bond is present in every known society, even in those that strive to deny its existence. They point out that toleration of plural marriage is not the same thing as actually living it. Most people around the world live out their lives within a monogamous union, with those inside a plural marriage often competing for their spouse's attention and hoping to become a "favorite" wife or husband. The strong pull toward emotional exclusivity suggests the impulse to form a pair bond is more relentless than poly advocates often prefer to acknowledge.

EQUAL OR RANKED LOVERS?

Research on polyamory indicates that it is difficult to sustain an "authentic" and "egalitarian" form of passionate plural love over time. No matter how relationships begin, most—though not all—polyamorous arrangements tend, within one to two years, to drift from an all-inclusive egalitarian union into a ranked love hierarchy featuring a primary partner and one or more secondary partners who may live either nearby or at a distance. For many practitioners, the more exclusive primary bond becomes the preferred love relationship. Primary partners typically spend the most time together, while secondary and tertiary partners—whose relationships often rest more on a generalized feeling of "liking," even when expressed as "love"—are valued as significant "others" but remain supplemental to the primary emotional connection.

As with many bisexual relationships, individuals frequently organize their emotional and physical spaces differently with each partner. More broadly, there appears to be an emotionally charged ranked preference: one sexual orientation tends to correspond to the primary lover, while the other orientation corresponds more to an affectionate and likeable sexual-emotional playmate.

Even with the adoption of pragmatic strategies designed to manage potentially disruptive emotions—such as maintaining geographical distance, a tactic widely used in plural love systems—jealousy remains a persistent potential source of conflict within polyamorous units. Researchers report that polyamorists, despite their philosophical embrace of loving multiple people simultaneously, are often engaged in an ongoing existential struggle to reconcile the desire for emotional abundance with the need for relational stability.

One frequent solution, as noted, is to rank-order partners, distributing attention and affection in proportion to one's emotional preference. In this regard, polyamory practitioners resemble polyandrous wives, who likewise rank husbands in terms of emotional closeness. The core difference lies in norms of disclosure: polyandrous wives usually prefer not to publicly acknowledge their rankings, whereas polyamory practitioners often consider open acknowledgment of ranked affection to be both honest and ethically important.

Perhaps most striking is the willingness of polyamorists to acknowledge shortcomings in their relationships, which they often view as a necessary step toward a higher ideal of honesty, emotional authenticity, and the possibility of more deeply felt love. Such aspirations are premised on open, reflective communication and an explicit willingness to confront relational difficulties.

By contrast, fundamentalist polygamous families are generally reluctant to acknowledge personal favoritism or emotional imbalance. Polygynous husbands are frequently overwhelmed by wives' complaints about insufficient material support or emotional reassurance. Yet for a man to publicly admit that his family has problems is to call into question his status as a successful provider and household manager—an identity failure that many men are deeply motivated to avoid.

POLYAMORY RESEARCH

Leanna Wolfe, who has conducted extensive research on polyamory, suggests that the polyamorous lifestyle holds particular appeal for "beta," or lower-status, men who are open to forming polyandrous-style arrangements—even if doing so means accepting a secondary-lover position (see Chapter 3 on the use of similar terminology within the "manosphere"). By contrast, "alpha," or higher-status, men tend to form polyfidelity units composed of one man and two women (preferably bisexual). To date, however, little research has verified, refined, or challenged this claim.

It is also difficult to know the distribution of different poly configurations. We suspect—but cannot be certain—that more men than women prefer "solo poly," and it remains unclear which form of poly coupling is most common: one woman with several men, one man with multiple women, or arrangements involving two or more women. Independent empirical research remains limited. Numerous online surveys report that polyamorists' life satisfaction is comparable to that of individuals in monogamous marriages, but these surveys do not inquire into participants' ideas about the experience of being in love.

Sheff's work remains one of the earliest and most comprehensive investigations. She finds wide variation in practitioners' motivations for participating in polyfidelity. Some participants are highly sexualized and embrace the lifestyle as a vehicle for justifying or fulfilling their desire for sexual variety. Others are asexual but seek richer, more emotionally fulfilling experiences than those they associate with monogamy. Still others, regardless of sexual drive, want to form and sustain an emotionally supportive bond with several familiars—even if doing so means they will never become a primary lover or pair bond partner.

Given practitioners' insistence on polyamory's superiority, why do so many eventually leave? Sheff's research—understandably lacking historical depth—cannot answer this question: the poly units she studied had not existed long enough to assess long-term stability. Earlier research, however, provides a suggestive baseline. Studies of "group marriages" (the terms *polyamory* and *polyamour* had not yet been coined) conducted in the 1960s found that these unions typically lasted no more than five years, with most dissolving after roughly 18 months. A five-year study of American "group marriage" conducted in the late 1960s found similar patterns. By contrast, monogamous marriages in the United States last, on average, between 15 and 22 years. Clearly, polyamory—despite its many celebrated virtues—has proven less sustainable. Why?

Sheff, like other researchers, identifies a persistent source of strain: the polyfidelity or "open" relationship ethos produces a chronic, often unvoiced, anxiety rooted in the fear of losing the primary lover's interest. The intensity of this fear varies across the life course. Younger practitioners, especially those in their reproductive years, tend to feel more threatened and exhibit stronger emotional responses. Individuals over 50 tend to have far milder reactions.

When jealousy emerges, practitioners typically blame themselves for their perceived shortcomings. A core axiom of polyamory holds that jealousy can and must be overcome, ideally through interpersonal dialogue that fosters emotional insight and personal growth. Most participants argue that jealousy should not be seen as an obstacle to developing a fuller and more meaningful form of plural love. Nonetheless, jealousy—whether voiced or unvoiced—remains a common emotional undercurrent. To counter it, practitioners first identify the triggers, then discuss their feelings with partners. In place of jealousy, they encourage the cultivation of *compersion* (see above)—the joy of knowing that one's partner has found another source of romantic happiness. This value is aspirational for some and a lived reality for others.

Yet when ordinary stresses accumulate, polyamorous relationships often prove harder to maintain than monogamous ones, especially when children are involved. As one polyamorist admitted, "To be honest, stress can kill poly love, along with the ordinary demands of living." Another added a frequent, not inaccurate, qualification: "Monogamy is not that great; I see failure everywhere too." Practitioners remain acutely aware of the tensions embedded in their lifestyle, just as they recognize the distinct, though different, tensions inherent in monogamy.

Here lies the dilemma: every family system carries its own built-in sources of strain as well as its own forms of heightened satisfaction. The challenge is to identify the system that best aligns with one's emotional, philosophical, and relational needs—a quest that, for many polyamorists, becomes a lifelong project. In an important sense, polyamory practitioners remain in a continuous dialogue with themselves and one another over the nature of love. Is there an underlying "essence" to love—one that might override personal philosophy or even preferred sexual orientation?

To approach such questions, we need more empirically grounded studies from diverse cultural contexts. To fully explore the social and emotional nuances of creating and sustaining a loving polyamorous relationship, it is instructive to examine the broader social and psychological complexities that Euro-Americans have long associated with being "in love."

WHAT IS LOVE?

If passionate or romantic love is organized around emotional exclusivity—requiring the reordering of an individual's motivational priorities—what happens when a person becomes emotionally (as opposed to primarily sexually) involved with more than one partner? We have already seen the difficulties that arise in polyandrous families (one wife with multiple husbands), polygynous families (one man with multiple wives), and now in polyamorous or "multiple-lover" relationships.

In one study of individuals who did not desire, and explicitly rejected, forming a polyfidelity bond yet nevertheless fell in love with two people at the same time, many initially reported little conflict. They attempted to balance both relationships through the creation of psychological and spatial boundaries—either by relying on geographical distance or by employing "psychological bracketing," a cognitive technique that allows them to mentally compartmentalize, at least temporarily, their involvement with another partner.

Several participants acknowledged experiencing what polyamorists often claim: a deeper, richer, and more meaningful sense of satisfaction when involved with multiple lovers. Clearly, some individuals have a capacity for sustaining deep, concurrent romantic attachments. Yet such arrangements seldom endure for significant periods. Over time, they tend to shift toward a companionship-based, rank-ordered form of plural love.

Every culture must confront the relationship between love and sex as these experiences are imagined, constructed, and lived. Because love—an intense emotional attachment—and sex—the desire for physical release—are often intertwined yet independent states, societies rarely allow unrestricted freedom for either impulse. Instead, cultures blend them in ways that support broader norms regarding kinship, inheritance, caste, class, gender, and theological principles.

We know that specific individuals can be lifelong sexually monogamous; we also know that humanity as a species is not. Sexual monogamy requires deliberate ethical commitment and sustained personal effort, raising a central question: Is it possible to be sexually libertine while remaining emotionally monogamous? This question lies at the heart of the polyamory lifestyle debate.

CONCLUSION

Cross-cultural research has demonstrated that passionate love is universal or near universal, sparking an expansion of ethnographic work that explores love across a wide range of societies. These studies document the cultural variability of romantic ideals and practices, challenging Euro-American assumptions about where and how "true love" ought to be expressed. This one partner becomes the preferred or primary attachment. This raises an intriguing question: Is the difficulty in sustaining egalitarian plural love the result of personality-specific traits that undermine one's earnest commitment to polyamory, or does it arise from a broader human difficulty in overriding deep-seated psychological and social norms favoring dyadic attachment?

We suspect that a small number of plural or poly-love relationships are indeed long-term, stable, and personally fulfilling. Yet ethnographic and historical studies consistently show such outcomes to be uncommon. Sociological analyses of plural or group-love arrangements repeatedly find that these relationships tend to confront insurmountable difficulties. Most are eventually abandoned in favor of a dyadic pair bond or a "primary/secondary" hierarchical emotional hierarchy.

We suggest that the problematic nature of polyfidelity arises from the dyadic organization of passionate love. While certain idiosyncratic polyamory relationships—such as Alexander Hamilton's long-term plural involvement with the Schuyler sisters—may be relatively successful, the historical and ethnographic record shows that such arrangements rarely scale up to a community level. Benjamin Zablocki's comprehensive sociological research likewise found that group-love arrangements were predictably fraught and, for most, ultimately untenable.

Clearly, some individuals possess the capacity to sustain deep, egalitarian, simultaneous loves. But when polyamorous bonds do endure, participants almost always develop strong companionship attachments that gradually evolve into an emotionally ranked hierarchy in which Even in Hamilton's well-known relationship with the Schuyler sisters, one sister emerged as his primary love while the other remained a valued but secondary romantic companion. The historical record thus mirrors the ethnographic pattern: egalitarian plural love is conceivable, occasionally attainable, but rarely sustainable.

The emergence of an emotional hierarchy in plural love relationships does not mean that participants do not "love" one another. Most do. Rather, it suggests that if plural love is to endure, it will be grounded more in companionship-based affection than in sustained passionate intensity. Ultimately, polyamorous or plural-love arrangements require deliberate effort—and often conscious determination—to maintain simultaneous and separate life histories or narratives. For many, this task becomes too demanding over time. The construction of distinct personae across relationships may also generate behaviors and attitudes reminiscent of a dual personality.

Regardless of how such behaviors are described, sustaining multiple personae often produces inner turmoil. These selves can be maintained temporarily, but typically at an emotional cost. The very goal participants hope to achieve may strain, or even fragment, their sense of self. As hopes erode under the pressure of divided emotional commitments, the foundation of the relationships they seek to nurture weakens as well. What begins as an attempt to satisfy passion, and secure companionship may devolve into a psychological dilemma experienced as deeply dissatisfying and ultimately self-destructive. The inability to merge passion and companionship into a stable whole underscores the primacy of the dyadic bond—a bond rooted more in emotional exclusivity than in sexual exclusivity. This emotional pull toward dyadic attachment challenges many polygynous, polyandrous, and polyamorous triadic arrangements.

Research on earlier plural-love communes likewise found that relatively few members reported genuine happiness, emotional fulfillment, or personal nourishment in their poly or plural-love relationships. These findings highlight the burdens entailed in departing from a pair bond model that, while sometimes uninspiring, provides emotional exclusivity and a sense of responsibility that many find stabilizing.

In sum, the impulse to form a pair bond is present—albeit in different proportions—in all societies, even in those that discourage emotional exclusivity, such as communities organized around arranged marriage, polygyny, or polyamory. Although both polygynous families and polyamory practitioners often justify their choices by asserting the superiority of plural love, these claims tend to rest more on aspiration than on demonstrated practice. Unlike monogamous marriages, polyamorous arrangements make it easier for participants to leave when the relationship no longer meets their expectations or needs. This dynamic aligns with many Euro-American millennials' reluctance to commit to long-term partnerships.

The aspirational efforts—and, for most, the eventual failure—to sustain polyamorous bonds of equal emotional intensity reveal a fundamental human condition shaped by two contradictory inclinations: the tendency toward sexual polygamy and the pull toward emotional monogamy. Across cultures, individuals must ultimately reconcile these competing behavioral and emotional orientations in their own lives.

FURTHER READING

Two works of fiction were significant in sparking explorations of "ethical non-monogamy" in the United States during the late twentieth century. Robert A. Heinlein's science fiction novel *Stranger in a Strange Land* (1961), though presenting an idealized and "impossible to live" model of group marriage, was a major source of inspiration for early intentional communities and groups like the Church of All Worlds that began experimenting with non-monogamy in the 1960s. Published a few years later, *The Harrad Experiment* (1966) by Robert H. Rimmer explored consensual non-monogamy in a contemporary, realistic setting, was influential among people considering alternative relationships during the late 1960s and early 1970s.

Two works of nonfiction written by polyamory advocates have also been important. *Loving More: The Polyfidelity Primer* (1992) by Ryam Nearing was written as a practical, foundational text that outlined polyfidelity (a closed form of non-monogamy) and provided guidelines for ethical non-monogamy. The author co-founded the *Loving More* magazine and organization, which became a primary vehicle for spreading polyamorous ideas. Clinical psychologist Deborah Anapol's *Love Without Limits* (1992, later reissued as *Polyamory: The New Love Without Limits* in 1997), provided a comprehensive framework that integrated psychological, spiritual, and mythic knowledge to define and advocate for polyamory. Her work helped to professionalize the discourse and establish the term "polyamory" as we know it today.

Finally, two more recent works of scholarly research stand out for their insights into polyamory's origins in the late twentieth century and its practice in the early twenty-first century. Sociologist Elisabeth Sheff's *The Polyamorists Next Door* (2013) offers an insider's view of life in polyamorous units. Using interviews and observations, the author followed hundreds of people, including children growing up in poly families. Historian Christopher Gleason's *American Poly: A History* (2023) is an accessible scholarly exploration of the origins of the polyamory lifestyle and movement in 1960s-era counterculture and neopaganism and of the movement's subsequent expansion.

BIBLIOGRAPHY

Anapol, D. (1997). *Polyamory: The new love without limits*. IntiNet Resource Center. (Original work published 1992.)

Gleason, C. (2023). *American poly: A history*. Oxford University Press.

Heinlein, R. A. (1961). *Stranger in a strange land*. G. P. Putnam's Sons.

Nearing, R. (1992). *Loving more: The polyfidelity primer*. IntiNet Resource Center.

Rimmer, R. H. (1966). *The Harrad experiment*. Sherbourne Press.

Sheff, E. (2013). *The polyamorists next door*. Rowman & Littlefield Publishers.

CONCLUSION

BEYOND THE MONOGAMOUS NUCLEAR FAMILY?

Margaret Mead, who could be considered America's greatest anthropologist and public intellectual of the twentieth century, wrote extensively about sex and family structure. Following the social and political tumult of the 1960s—a time when many young Americans experimented with various forms of sexual and intimate relationships—Mead wrote: "No matter how many communes anybody invents, the family always creeps back."

Mead was no defender of the social status quo, however. She believed that marriage had become far too central in American society of the late twentieth century (which she described as "terribly over-married"), and she often assailed the restrictive nature of the monogamous nuclear family, particularly for women. She yearned for a future American society in which marriage and parenthood were simply among the options available to women, rather than exclusive preconditions of their full membership in society.

Is it possible to imagine a future, in the United States and other countries where monogamy has long been the only legally recognized and socially legitimized form of marriage, in which monogamy is simply one among many marital options? Our exploration of the place of plural marriage in the human experience might suggest a few answers to this question.

DOI: 10.4324/9781003628729-9

POLYGAMY'S MYTHS AND REALITIES

Plural marriage is no evolutionary anomaly in the story of humanity. Rather, it has long been an integral feature of many human societies. While some forms, most notably polyandry, have been historically rare, others, particularly polygyny, appear across a very wide range of cultural and geographic contexts. Throughout this book, we have highlighted both areas of disagreement and convergence within the scientific and historical literature on plural marriage. In this concluding chapter, we revisit these debates and reflect on polygamy's place in human affairs. We begin by reviewing some of the myths about polygamy that research can refute.

Polygamy has long evoked both fascination and repulsion among people living in societies where it is not practiced openly or widely. Over time, several persistent myths have shaped popular and scholarly understandings of the practice. The first and perhaps most dangerous myth is that plural marriage has always been the exception to the rule. This belief is rooted in the assumption that humans are naturally monogamous and that monogamy represents our evolutionary "default." As we have shown, plural marriage has existed across an extraordinarily diverse array of societies and continues to thrive in many today. In some contexts, it has been restricted to elites; in others, it has been broadly accessible. Given the cross-cultural and historical record, we must reject the notion that humans are somehow "hard-wired" exclusively for monogamy.

This conclusion does not imply, however, that monogamy is "unnatural" for our species. Indeed, we would do well to abandon the language of "natural" versus "unnatural" altogether when discussing marriage systems. Nor should we assume that either monogamy or polygamy is inherently superior. In many societies, monogamous marriage is experienced as a rewarding—if sometimes challenging—institution that supports individuals' life goals. In other cultural settings, polygamy fulfills a similar role, functioning as a socially legitimate system that aligns with prevailing economic, reproductive, and familial priorities.

A second enduring myth stems from popular fascination with the "Orientalist" polygamous family, particularly in Middle Eastern contexts. This image, shaped by colonial imagination and popular media, portrays polygamy as an exoticized fantasy characterized by sexual excess and the subjugation of women. Similar narratives were later applied to nineteenth-century Mormon polygamy, where outsiders often depicted women as "slaves" to men's unrestrained sexual desires. Ethnographic and comparative research across diverse societies, however, consistently challenges these portrayals.

Polygamous families are typically organized around reproduction, household labor, and the long-term care of women and children, rather than sexual gratification. Sexual access is generally understood as secondary to reproductive and familial responsibilities. Far from being a system designed primarily for male pleasure, polygamy entails substantial material, emotional, and organizational demands. When practiced seriously, it constitutes a complex family system structured around the needs and obligations of wives, mothers, and children, and embedded within broader moral, economic, and social frameworks.

A third myth, an especially persistent and pernicious one, concerns the relationship between polygyny and young single men. In Chapter 5, we reviewed the research in political science highlighting a strong association between polygyny and violence: societies with high rates of polygynous marriage tend to face higher risks of violence in many forms, from domestic abuse at the household level to civil wars at the national level. The existence of such an association is beyond dispute. The problem is that the nature of this association is not as clear as some scholars have made it out to be, mainly because of the issue of single men's access to marriage markets. To infer that widespread polygyny must exclude significant numbers of young men from the marriage market is logical, even commonsensical; surely, this logic goes, whenever one man takes multiple wives, another man is condemned to bachelorhood.

But this inference, logical as it may be, is based on two erroneous assumptions about sex ratios and marriage markets. The first is that the numbers of male and female participants in the marriage market must not be significantly different. The second is that males experience their delayed entry into marriage as a form of generational oppression. Decades of demographic and ethnographic research on high-polygyny societies all over the world, particularly in sub-Saharan Africa, challenge both assumptions. As we saw in Chapter 3, the data show that such societies are characterized by much higher rates of male marriage than are most other societies around the globe; in fact, male marriage rates in high-polygyny African contexts verge on universal. One place where we *do* find young men shut out of the marriage market in polygynous communities is among fundamentalist Mormons in the United States, a setting where few would likely blame a propensity for political violence and instability on plural marriage. The notion that polygyny generally radicalizes young men by diminishing their marriage prospects does not stand up to scientific scrutiny.

Rather than viewing polygyny as a root cause of violence, it would be more helpful to understand it as a proxy for patriarchy, misogyny, and gender inequality (which together help compose the Patriarchal/Fraternal Syndrome described by Hudson and colleagues, discussed in Chapter 5). Where these forces are strong, women and girls have highly restricted autonomy, circumscribed mobility, and limited choice over marriage. If we presume that, all things being equal, most women would prefer not to share their husbands with other women (and there is ample evidence to support this presumption), then rather than interpreting a high prevalence of polygynous marriages as evidence that women are acting on an imperative to choose the "fittest" husbands, we should conclude that compared to men, women have reduced agency in the marriage market and fewer good options to choose from. Research suggests that more women enter polygynous marriages out of a lack of better alternatives than out of a preference for, as George Bernard Shaw put it, "a tenth share in a first-rate man."

POLYGYNY AND HUMAN NATURE: ONGOING DEBATES

At present, there is lively disagreement among scholars regarding the significance of the human pair bond. Constructionist perspectives view pair bonding primarily as a product of social and cultural forces designed to promote cooperation rather than as an evolved biological imperative. From this perspective, monogamy is not the result of innate human design but of historically contingent norms and institutions. As anthropologist Agustín Fuentes argues, "We can be monogamous, but our bodies and minds are not specifically designed for it." Other constructionists further suggest that monogamy represents a relatively recent behavioral development in *Homo sapiens*, emerging from shifts in economic organization and social regulation rather than from our species' evolutionary foundations.

Evolutionary perspectives, by contrast, locate pair bonding more firmly within human biology and psychology. From this view, the impulse to form strong, selective, and enduring emotional attachments is deeply rooted in the human condition and plays a critical role in child-rearing, family stability, and social order. For evolutionists, the persistence of polygamy across history does not negate the pair bond; rather, it represents a social arrangement that exists alongside—and sometimes in tension with—the underlying pull toward dyadic attachment. In the debate between constructionists and evolutionists, no resolution appears to be on the horizon.

Another debate concerns the evolutionary advantages or disadvantages conferred by polygamy. Certainly, in some specific cultural and geographical settings, polygyny or polyandry might constitute practices that enable households to cooperate better and to adapt more efficiently to their environment. Likewise, in some settings—most notably polygynous ones—having multiple wives allows for larger families and therefore more domestic or agricultural labor. Yet these advantages are highly context-specific. We observed in Chapter 3 that neither in human reproduction nor economic production does polygyny confer any general, consistent advantages, and that only from the perspective of husbands (not wives) can polygyny constitute an asset with respect to numbers of offspring—but even this observation is qualified by the role of child mortality, which seems to be higher in some polygynous communities relative to their monogamous neighbors.

As we saw in Chapter 5, some scholars have portrayed polygyny as inherently maladaptive, oppressive to women, and requiring abolition. Leaving aside the many practical concerns over how abolition could be achieved, their arguments frequently rest on weak foundations, such as the idea that polygyny prevents large numbers of men from marrying. Yet those who defend polygyny have often done so on traditional or identitarian grounds, framing plural marriage as a way to connect with putatively "pure" ancestral cultures (particularly in African and Middle Eastern settings and diasporas). Disagreements about polygyny are unlikely to be resolved, for they tend to be driven more by political than scientific motives.

BUT ISN'T MONOGAMY STILL BETTER THAN POLYGAMY?

At this point, some readers may be wondering: Why doesn't this concluding chapter just declare that monogamy is the superior marital form? Haven't the preceding chapters offered ample evidence of this? We saw in Chapter 2 that polygyny imposes high costs on the psychological and physical health of men, women, and children. We saw in Chapter 3 that due to the very real threats of conflict and household resource dilution, most women prefer not to have to share their husbands with other wives. We saw in Chapter 6 that polyandry poses problems of its own. Why not simply conclude that monogamy is what's best for everyone?

These are valid questions. The mistake we want to avoid, however, is "comparing the worst kinds of polygyny with the ideal kinds of monogamy," in the words of political scientist Ronald Den Otter. From Salt Lake City to Senegal to Sumatra, many of the most serious problems faced in polygynous households stem less from inherent aspects of plural marriage and more from broader systemic factors such as sexism, patriarchy, and especially poverty. The ideal forms of monogamy against which many Western readers compare instances of polygamy—monogamy in which both partners are sexually faithful, husbands do not abuse their wives, and everyone has enough agency and resources to meet their basic needs—is probably no more realistic than the ideal forms of polygamy that many advocates of plural marriage hold up to argue the inferiority of monogamy. We must always bear in mind that monogamous marriages can be "high functioning" and "low functioning," just as polygynous marriages can (see Chapter 4).

Which type of marriage is "best" depends entirely on the reader's judgment of what marriage is supposed to be, or perhaps of what its "function" is. As we argued in Chapter 3, such a judgment flows not from empirical, scientific knowledge but from cultural standards. A monogamous marriage may be better than a polygynous one at fostering the conditions in which spouses can develop deep attachments based on trust and emotional intimacy. On the other hand, a polygynous marriage may be better than a monogamous one at fostering the conditions in which members of a large household can thrive and help reproduce their lineage in conditions of economic uncertainty. Whether you prefer polygamy or monogamy depends on many factors, not least among which is what you value most in marriage and in life.

WHAT FUTURE FOR POLYGYNY, POLYAMORY, AND MONOGAMY?

As we saw in Chapter 7, the legal and cultural landscape pertaining to marriage and sexuality has shifted rapidly in the United States and many other countries since the beginning of this century. The right of homosexual couples to marry, which seemed either unthinkable or unattainable to many people only a few years ago, has become enshrined in law in more than three dozen countries. It is possible to imagine, as some opponents of same-sex marriage have, a not-too-distant future in which plural marriage enjoys similar legal recognition in lands where it has long been illegal, clandestine, and shunned. Polyamory, likewise, has gone from a little-known practice in a few "alternative communities" to an aspiration widely shared by young people in wealthy countries. It is also possible therefore to imagine a future in which poly families exist openly, proudly, and legally.

Social conservatives and even some polyamorists see in such a future the inevitable doom of monogamous marriage. While monogamy will probably continue its decline in these countries, however, we think it is too early to count it out. The study of polygamous and polyamorous relationships suggests, at the very least, that an exclusive and durable sexual relationship is something that many people require and will continue to demand. As polyamory continues its shift out of the circumscribed realm of communal movements and intentional communities and into the cultural mainstream, it will appeal to growing numbers of educated, urban individuals who are wary of emotionally exclusive relationships. We cannot yet say how well established it might become.

As for polygyny, it is unlikely to become widespread in wealthy societies in which women enjoy significant legal rights, such as the United States. We have seen that its prevalence today is greatest in impoverished societies lacking gender equality, either in law or in social norms. Wherever women have greater agency and a determining say over their future, polygyny will remain an unattractive option for most of them. And in societies where it is already practiced, particularly in the Islamic world and in sub-Saharan Africa, polygyny is already becoming something of an elite privilege as urbanization raises its associated economic costs. In many fast-growing cities, polygynous marriages have transitioned from complex, single households to dispersed, multilocal households—at least for those fortunate enough to be able to afford them. As noted at the end of Chapter 4, this transition is already transforming the local meaning of kinship and the nature of relations between and among co-wives as well as half-siblings. For less well-off individuals in these cities, formal polygyny may be unaffordable, but informal variations of it (along the lines of existing roles such as "outside wives" and "second offices") offer similar alternatives. In urban Senegal, the figure of the *mbaraan*—a woman with multiple informal male partners—has become a newfangled (if informal and still officially illicit) kind of polyandry; it fits into broader West African patterns in which women cultivate co-parental ties with multiple fathers of their children.

Finally, what future exists for monogamy? Its practice has certainly diminished in recent decades and is almost certain to continue diminishing for decades more. Our review of the historical and ethnographic research demonstrates that significant portions of humanity have long considered that monogamy does not help them meet their material or emotional needs. And yet, we do not foresee monogamy's demise: it has been the dominant form of marriage for thousands of years, and we think it will retain that status. For all its challenges and shortcomings, for all the dissatisfaction, cheating, and experimentation to which it gives rise, monogamy seems to fulfill certain deep-seated human needs. Theories about the pair bond fail to explain all human sexual or marital behavior; they cannot account for the high prevalence of sexual infidelity and extra-pair fertility. But they do suggest that most humans will continue to seek out exclusive emotional and sexual relationships, and will maintain those relationships (however imperfectly) for as long as they can.

WHY DO PEOPLE SEE THE PAIR BOND AS SOMETHING OF A DOWNER?

Across cultures and historical epochs, human beings display a marked tendency toward pair bonding. Even in societies that formally discourage emotional exclusivity—through arranged marriage, polygyny, or polyamory—individuals routinely gravitate toward a primary attachment. This persistence suggests that pair bonding is not merely a cultural artifact but a human propensity. Yet this preference raises a paradox: if the pair bond is so deeply rooted, why do so many people repeatedly reject it in favor of alternative forms of intimate life? What accounts for the enduring appeal of plural love?

One answer lies in the promise of expanded possibility. Plural love appeals to the intuition that human connection need not be confined to a single dyadic structure. If life satisfaction is shaped by the richness and density of our relational world, then restricting our most intimate bonds to one person may feel unnecessarily limiting. The dyad, for all its emotional power, can seem to narrow the field of human significance rather than enlarge it. Plural love offers an imagined abundance: more intimacy, more understanding, more erotic vitality, and more mirrors through which the self may be seen and affirmed.

This appeal is not merely pragmatic; it is deeply imaginative. Human beings possess an extraordinary capacity to envision alternative worlds and to experience dissatisfaction with the one they inhabit. The yearning to transcend the dyadic bond arises from this imaginative faculty, coupled with the desire for more complex and encompassing forms of love. Plural love thus becomes a site where the human longing for novelty, expansion, and transformation converges with erotic and emotional aspiration. It is not only a different arrangement of relationships, but a different vision of what love itself might be.

Closely intertwined with this vision is a utopian impulse. Plural love is often imagined as a communal ideal—an arrangement capable of meeting more needs, satisfying more desires, and dissolving the constraints imposed by exclusivity. It promises a form of emotional plenitude in which no single relationship bears the full burden of meaning. In this sense, plural love functions as a secular form of transcendence. Where religious traditions once offered union with the divine, plural love offers fusion with an idealized network of intimacy. It becomes a vehicle for personal enlightenment, a path toward a more expansive and emotionally intensified mode of being.

This utopian promise helps explain why plural love is periodically reinvented by each generation, adorned with new metaphors, ethical frameworks, and claims to truth. Whether framed as liberation, authenticity, or emotional evolution, it is repeatedly offered as an answer to the perceived limitations of conventional romantic life. The dream persists because it speaks to a fundamental human desire: not merely to love, but to love more fully, more intensely, and more meaningfully.

And yet, despite its enduring appeal, plural love proves remarkably difficult to sustain in actual practice. The difficulty lies not in social stigma alone, but in a deeper psychological tension. Pair bonding excels at providing emotional security, predictability, and attachment stability. Plural love, by contrast, amplifies uncertainty, comparison, and vulnerability. Even when participants consciously reject exclusivity, patterns of hierarchy and preference often reassert themselves. Competition for attention resurfaces, jealousy reemerges under new rationalizations, and informal dyads quietly form within the larger structure.

What plural love seeks to overcome—the limitations of the pair bond—it often ends up reproducing in subtler form. The longing for transcendence collides with the equally powerful need for security. Human beings appear to desire both relational abundance and emotional anchoring, yet these desires operate according to different and often incompatible logics.

The persistent failure of plural love, then, should not be understood simply as personal weakness or cultural resistance. Rather, it reflects a constitutive tension within human intimacy itself. We are creatures who crave stability and transformation, attachment and expansion, belonging and transcendence. The pair bond satisfies some of these longings, plural love others, but no single arrangement resolves them all.

Plural love endures as a dream not because it is easily realized, but because it gives form to what the pair bond cannot fully contain. It represents the human refusal to accept finitude in love, even as experience repeatedly teaches its necessity. In this oscillation between security and transcendence, between the dyad and its imagined alternatives, the history of human intimacy continues to unfold.

INDEX

For Product Safety Concerns and Information please contact our EU representative GPSR@taylorandfrancis.com
Taylor & Francis Verlag GmbH, Kaufingerstraße 24, 80331 München, Germany

www.ingramcontent.com/pod-product-compliance
Lightning Source LLC
LaVergne TN
LVHW021300151026
850117LV00030B/307
* 9 7 8 1 0 4 1 0 4 5 4 2 7 *